Anatomical Atlas of Acupuncture Points

About the Author

Yan Zhenguo graduated in 1956 as Bachelor of Medicine from the Medical School of
Qi Lu University in Shandong, one of China's oldest and most respected universities. Since
then he has worked in the Anatomy Department of the Shanghai University of Traditional
Chinese Medicine. He obtained a Ph.D. in medicine at the Medical School of Osaka
University (Japan) in 1982 and was appointed Professor of Shanghai University of
Traditional Chinese Medicine in 1986.

    Professor Yan is a supervisor of Ph.D. and postdoctoral students and visiting researcher at
the Medical School of Osaka University. He is also a regular lecturer at Hong Kong
University.

    Professor Yan is a pioneer of the anatomy of acupuncture points in China and has received
numerous awards for his achievements. He has published many books, atlases and articles
and is chief editor of the Textbook of Anatomy for Traditional Chinese Medicine. Many of his
books have been translated and published in English, Japanese, French, German, Spanish,
Russian, and Arabic.

ANATOMICAL ATLAS OF ACUPUNCTURE POINTS

Written by
Yan Zhenguo
Professor, Shanghai University of Traditional Chinese Medicine

Editorial Committee
**Yan Zhenguo, Zhang Jianhua, Shao Shuijin, Zhao Yingxia,
Zhang Xuexiang, Zhang Liancai**

Illustrations
Chen Tingli, Li Chengjian, Yan Wei, Yang Lida

Photographs
Xie Lin, Song Zhiqun

Model
Zhuo Huifang

English Supervisor
Li Zhaoguo

Translators
Wei Hai, Yan Zhenguo

Subject editor
Trina Ward MPhil, BSc (Hons), MRCHM, MBAcC

Medical consultant
Dr. Robert J. Dickie FRCGP, DRCOG, BMedBiol

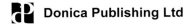 Donica Publishing Ltd

Note

Medical knowledge is constantly changing. As new information becomes available, changes in treatment, procedures, equipment and techniques become necessary. The editors/authors/contributors and the publishers have, as far as it is possible, taken care to ensure that the information given in this text is accurate and up to date. However, readers are strongly advised to confirm that the information complies with the latest legislation and standards of practice.

Although every effort has been made to indicate appropriate precautions with regard to the acupuncture points discussed in this book, neither the publishers nor the authors can accept responsibility for any treatment advice or information offered, neither will they be liable for any loss or damage of any nature occasioned to or suffered by any person acting or refraining from acting as a result of reliance on the material contained in this publication.

First published 2003

ISBN 1 901149 05 6

British Library Cataloguing in Publication Data
A catalogue record for this book is available from the British Library

Commissioning editor Yanping Li
Managing editor Rodger Watts
Cover design Paul Robinson

Typeset and printed in China.
The publisher's policy is to use paper manufactured from sustainable forests.

Preface

This *Anatomical Atlas of Acupuncture Points* offers a large selection of color photographs illustrating the location of acupuncture points and channels in relation to the anatomic structure of the human body. Treatment by acupuncture and moxibustion achieves its effect through needling or warming acupuncture points on the body surface to dredge the channels and regulate Qi and Blood. Correct location of acupuncture points and familiarity with the anatomic structures related to the needle passage is therefore the key to the therapeutic effect of these treatment methods.

This book is essentially divided into three sections. The first section provides full-color photographs of the location of the main acupuncture channels and their points superimposed on a human model. A "cascade" structure leads from whole body views through location by channel to regional and local views. The second section shows cross-sectional anatomic views of the main acupuncture points located on the trunk, enabling all the main internal structures to be related to these points.

The third section offers a selection of commonly used or potentially more dangerous acupuncture points, illustrating the needle passage in photographs and diagrams and highlighting structures to be avoided. In addition, this section also provides details of the physical location of the points, needling techniques and insertion methods, actions and indications, stratified anatomy, and appropriate cautions.

For many years, I have been engaged in the study of the sectional and stratified anatomy of acupuncture points, CT scintigrams of these points, and their microstructure and stereoscopic structure. This involves a multi-disciplinary approach, incorporating the integration of Western medicine and Traditional Chinese Medicine as well as theoretical research and clinical practice. The results of some of my research, based on the application of computed tomography (CT) scans to acupuncture points, is detailed in a brief appendix.

This atlas is compiled in accordance with the Acupuncture Points Schedule included in the National Acupuncture Points Standard of the People's Republic of China issued by the State Bureau of Technical Supervision in September 1990 and published by the State Standardization Press. I also participated in the Study on Acupuncture Points and their Anatomic Structure organized by the State Administrative Bureau of Traditional Chinese Medicine and the results of the study are incorporated in this book.

This atlas is intended as an aid for practicing acupuncturists and for teachers and students at TCM colleges around the world to assist in the accurate location of points and to increase needling confidence. It is my hope that this book will encourage more students to take up acupuncture to enable its benefits to be passed on to their patients.

Yan Zhenguo
Shanghai, June 2003

Contents

1 General figures of acupuncture points   1

FIGURES OF ACUPUNCTURE POINTS,
ANATOMICAL AND STANDING POSTURES   1
Anterior aspect acupuncture points, anatomical
posture   1
Posterior aspect acupuncture points, anatomical
posture   2
Anterior aspect acupuncture points, standing
posture   3
Posterior aspect acupuncture points, standing
posture   4
Left lateral aspect acupuncture points, standing
posture   5
Right lateral aspect acupuncture points, standing
posture   6

FIGURES OF ACUPUNCTURE POINTS, CASUAL
POSTURE   7
Points on the Lung and Heart channels   7
Points on the Large Intestine and Bladder
channels   8
Large Intestine and Bladder channel points on the
head and neck   9
Points on the Stomach and Pericardium
channels   10
Points on the Spleen and Liver channels   11
Points on the Small Intestine and Triple Burner
channels   12
Points on the Kidney channel and Conception
vessel   13
Points on the Gallbladder channel   14
Points on the Gallbladder channel (lateral aspect of
the head and neck)   15
Points on the Governor vessel   16
Governor vessel points on the head   17

2 Regional figures of acupuncture points   19

FIGURES OF ACUPUNCTURE POINTS ON THE
TRUNK   19
Acupuncture points, anterior aspect of the
trunk   19
Acupuncture points, posterior aspect of the
trunk   20

Acupuncture points, left lateral aspect of the
trunk   21
Acupuncture points, right lateral aspect of the
trunk   22
Acupuncture points, anterior aspect of the chest   23
Acupuncture points on the abdomen   24
Acupuncture points on the back   25
Acupuncture points on the lumbosacral region   26
Acupuncture points, lateral aspect of the chest   27
Acupuncture points, lateral aspect of the hip   28
Extraordinary acupuncture points on the
abdomen   29
Acupuncture points on the perineum   30

FIGURES OF ACUPUNCTURE POINTS ON THE
HEAD AND NECK   31
Acupuncture points, anterior aspect of the head and
neck   31
Acupuncture points, posterior aspect of the head
and neck   32
Acupuncture points, left lateral aspect of the head
and neck   33
Acupuncture points, right lateral aspect of the head
and neck   34
Acupuncture points on the vertex   35
Acupuncture points, anterior aspect of the neck   36

FIGURES OF ACUPUNCTURE POINTS ON THE ARM
AND HAND   37
Acupuncture points, anterior aspect of the arm and
hand   37
Acupuncture points, posterior aspect of the arm
and hand   37
Acupuncture points, radial aspect of the arm and
hand   38
Acupuncture points, ulnar aspect of the arm and
hand   38
Acupuncture points in the axillary region   39
Acupuncture points, anteromedial aspect of the
arm and hand   40
Acupuncture points, anterior aspect of the upper
arm   41
Acupuncture points, posterior aspect of the upper
arm   41

Acupuncture points, anterior aspect of the upper arm   42

Acupuncture points, anterior aspect of the forearm   43

Acupuncture points, posterior aspect of the forearm   43

Acupuncture points, anterior aspect of the forearm   44

Acupuncture points, posteromedial aspect of the hand   44

Acupuncture points on the palm   45

Acupuncture points on the dorsum of the hand   46

FIGURES OF ACUPUNCTURE POINTS ON THE LEG AND FOOT   47

Acupuncture points, anterior aspect of the leg and foot   47

Acupuncture points, posterior aspect of the leg and foot   48

Acupuncture points, medial aspect of the leg and foot   49

Acupuncture points, lateral aspect of the leg and foot   50

Acupuncture points, anterior aspect of the thigh   51

Acupuncture points, posterior aspect of the thigh   52

Acupuncture points, anteromedial aspect of the thigh   53

Acupuncture points, lateral aspect of the thigh   54

Acupuncture points, anterior aspect of the lower leg   55

Acupuncture points, posterior aspect of the lower leg   55

Acupuncture points, medial aspect of the lower leg   56

Acupuncture points, lateral aspect of the lower leg   56

Acupuncture points on the dorsum of the foot   57

Acupuncture points on the sole of the foot   57

Acupuncture points, medial aspect of the foot   58

Acupuncture points, lateral aspect of the foot   58

EAR ACUPUNCTURE POINTS   59

Acupuncture points on the anterior lateral side of the auricle   59

Acupuncture points on the dorsum of the auricle   60

3 Acupuncture points (sagittal section, left side)   61

Conception and Governor vessel points on the head, neck and trunk   61

Conception and Governor vessel points on the upper trunk   62

Conception and Governor vessel points on the lower trunk   63

Abdominal points on the Kidney channel, 0.5 cun lateral to the anterior midline   64

Kidney channel points on the upper trunk, 0.5 cun lateral to the anterior midline   65

Kidney channel points on the lower trunk, 0.5 cun lateral to the anterior midline   66

Points on the Kidney and Stomach channels, 2 cun lateral to the anterior midline   67

Kidney channel points on the chest, 2 cun lateral to the anterior midline   68

Stomach channel points on the abdomen, 2 cun lateral to the anterior midline   69

Points on the Stomach and Spleen channels, 4 cun lateral to the anterior midline   70

Stomach channel points on the chest, 4 cun lateral to the anterior midline   71

Spleen channel points on the abdomen, 4 cun lateral to the anterior midline   72

Points on the Bladder channel, 1.5 cun lateral to the posterior midline   73

Bladder channel points on the upper back, 1.5 cun lateral to the posterior midline   74

Bladder channel points on the lower back, 1.5 cun lateral to the posterior midline   75

Points on the Bladder channel, 3 cun lateral to the posterior midline   76

Bladder channel points on the upper back, 3 cun lateral to the posterior midline   77

Bladder channel points on the lower back, 3 cun lateral to the posterior midline   78

4 Sectional figures of acupuncture points on the head, neck and trunk   79

ACUPUNCTURE POINTS ON THE HEAD AND NECK   79

BL-1 Jingming, transverse sectional figure   79

GB-3 Shangguan, transverse sectional figure   80

Bitong, transverse sectional figure   81

LI-20 Yingxiang, transverse sectional figure 82
EX-HN-14 Yiming, transverse sectional figure   83
ST-4 Dicang, transverse sectional figure   84
GV-16 Fengfu and GB-20 Fengchi, transverse
sectional figure   85
SI-17 Tianrong, transverse sectional figure   86
CV-23 Lianquan, transverse sectional figure   87
ST-9 Renying and LI-18 Futu, transverse sectional
figure   88
ST-1 Chengqi and ST-2 Sibai, sagittal sectional
figure   89

ACUPUNCTURE POINTS ON THE TRUNK   91
LU-2 Yunmen, transverse sectional figure   91
CV-22 Tiantu, transverse sectional figure   92
ST-14 Kufang, transverse sectional figure   93
SP-20 Zhourong, transverse sectional figure   94
KI-25 Shencang, transverse sectional figure   95
ST-16 Yingchuang, transverse sectional figure   96
CV-17 Danzhong, transverse sectional figure   97
KI-22 Bulang, transverse sectional figure   98
CV-15 Jiuwei, transverse sectional figure   99
CV-14 Juque, transverse sectional figure   100
CV-13 Shangwan, transverse sectional figure   101
CV-12 Zhongwan, transverse sectional figure   102
CV-11 Jianli, transverse sectional figure   103
CV-10 Xiawan, transverse sectional figure   104
CV-9 Shuifen, transverse sectional figure   105
ST-25 Tianshu, transverse sectional figure   106
CV-7 Yinjiao, transverse sectional figure   107
CV-6 Qihai, transverse sectional figure   108
CV-5 Shimen, transverse sectional figure   109
CV-4 Guanyuan, transverse sectional figure   110
CV-3 Zhongji, transverse sectional figure   111
CV-2 Qugu, transverse sectional figure   112
GV-14 Dazhui, transverse and sagittal sectional
figures   113
BL-13 Feishu, transverse and sagittal sectional
figures   114
BL-14 Jueyinshu, transverse and sagittal sectional
figures   115
BL-15 Xinshu, transverse and sagittal sectional
figures   116
BL-16 Dushu, transverse and sagittal sectional
figures   117
BL-17 Geshu, transverse and sagittal sectional
figures   118

EX-B-3 Weiwanxiashu, transverse and sagittal
sectional figures   119
BL-18 Ganshu, transverse and sagittal sectional
figures   120
BL-19 Danshu, transverse and sagittal sectional
figures   121
BL-20 Pishu, transverse and sagittal sectional
figures   122
BL-21 Weishu, transverse and sagittal sectional
figures   123
BL-22 Sanjiaoshu, transverse and sagittal sectional
figures   124
BL-23 Shenshu, transverse and sagittal sectional
figures   125
BL-24 Qihaishu, transverse and sagittal sectional
figures   126
BL-25 Dachangshu, transverse and sagittal sectional
figures   127
BL-26 Guanyuanshu, transverse and sagittal
sectional figures   128
BL-31 Shangliao, transverse sectional figure 129
BL-32 Ciliao, transverse sectional figure   130
BL-33 Zhongliao, transverse sectional figure 131
BL-34 Xialiao, transverse and sagittal sectional
figures   132
GV-1 Changqiang, transverse and sagittal sectional
figures   133

5 Sectional figures of acupuncture points on the limbs   135

ACUPUNCTURE POINTS ON THE ARM AND
HAND   135
LI-15 Jianyu, sagittal sectional figure   135
LU-4 Xiabai, transverse sectional figure   136
LU-5 Chize, transverse sectional figure   137
LI-10 Shousanli, transverse sectional figure   138
LI-9 Shanglian, transverse sectional figure   139
LI-8 Xialian, transverse sectional figure   140
LU-6 Kongzui, transverse sectional figure   141
Bizhong, transverse sectional figure   142
PC-4 Ximen, transverse sectional figure   143
EX-UE-2 Erbai, transverse sectional figure   144
PC-5 Jianshi, transverse sectional figure   145
PC-6 Neiguan, transverse sectional figure   146
LU-7 Lieque, transverse sectional figure   147

HT-5 Tongli, transverse sectional figure   148
HT-6 Yinxi, transverse sectional figure   149
HT-7 Shenmen, transverse sectional figure   150
SI-4 Wangu, transverse sectional figure   151
LU-10 Yuji, transverse sectional figure   152
LI-4 Hegu, transverse sectional figure   153
PC-8 Laogong, transverse sectional figure   154

ACUPUNCTURE POINTS ON THE LEG AND FOOT 155
GB-30 Huantiao, transverse sectional figure   155
LR-11 Yinlian, transverse sectional figure   156
BL-36 Chengfu, transverse sectional figure   157
BL-37 Yinmen, transverse sectional figure   158
GB-31 Fengshi, transverse sectional figure   159
ST-32 Futu, transverse sectional figure   160
SP-10 Xuehai, transverse sectional figure   161
GB-34 Yanglingquan, transverse sectional figure   162
EX-LE-6 Dannang, transverse sectional figure   163
ST-36 Zusanli, transverse sectional figure   164
EX-LE-7 Lanwei, transverse sectional figure   165

ST-37 Shangjuxu, transverse sectional figure   166
ST-40 Fenglong, transverse sectional figure   167
KI-9 Zhubin, transverse sectional figure   168
GB-37 Guangming, transverse sectional figure   169
SP-6 Sanyinjiao, transverse sectional figure   170
KI-7 Fuliu, transverse sectional figure   171
ST-41 Jiexi, transverse sectional figure   172
SP-5 Shangqiu, transverse sectional figure   173
LR-3 Taichong, transverse sectional figure   174

Appendix   Computed tomography (CT) scan of acupuncture points   175
CT scan of LI-20 Yingxiang and SI-18 Quanliao   176
CT scan of LI-18 Futu and SI-16 Tianchuang   177
CT scan of LU-1 Zhongfu   178
CT scan of LI-4 Hegu   179
CT scan of GB-30 Huantiao   180
CT scan of ST-36 Zusanli   181

Index   183

1 General figures of acupuncture points

FIGURES OF ACUPUNCTURE POINTS, ANATOMICAL AND STANDING POSTURES

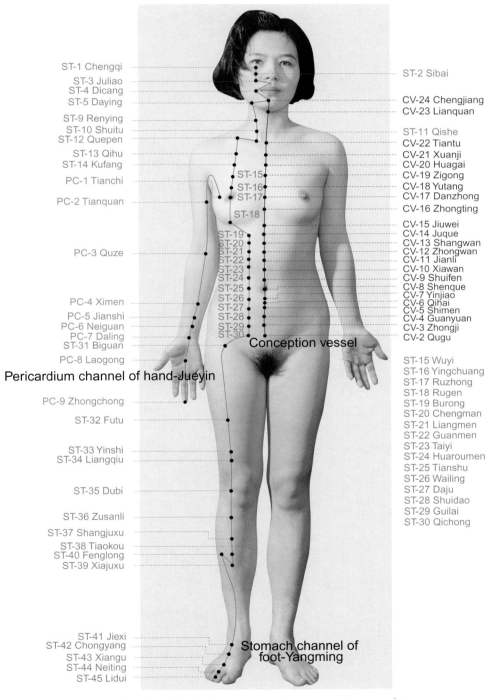

ST-1 Chengqi
ST-3 Juliao
ST-4 Dicang
ST-5 Daying
ST-9 Renying
ST-10 Shuitu
ST-12 Quepen
ST-13 Qihu
ST-14 Kufang
PC-1 Tianchi
PC-2 Tianquan
PC-3 Quze
PC-4 Ximen
PC-5 Jianshi
PC-6 Neiguan
PC-7 Daling
ST-31 Biguan
PC-8 Laogong

Pericardium channel of hand-Jueyin

PC-9 Zhongchong
ST-32 Futu
ST-33 Yinshi
ST-34 Liangqiu
ST-35 Dubi
ST-36 Zusanli
ST-37 Shangjuxu
ST-38 Tiaokou
ST-40 Fenglong
ST-39 Xiajuxu
ST-41 Jiexi
ST-42 Chongyang
ST-43 Xiangu
ST-44 Neiting
ST-45 Lidui

ST-15
ST-16
ST-17
ST-18
ST-19
ST-20
ST-21
ST-22
ST-23
ST-24
ST-25
ST-26
ST-27
ST-28
ST-29
ST-30

Conception vessel

ST-2 Sibai
CV-24 Chengjiang
CV-23 Lianquan
ST-11 Qishe
CV-22 Tiantu
CV-21 Xuanji
CV-20 Huagai
CV-19 Zigong
CV-18 Yutang
CV-17 Danzhong
CV-16 Zhongting
CV-15 Jiuwei
CV-14 Juque
CV-13 Shangwan
CV-12 Zhongwan
CV-11 Jianli
CV-10 Xiawan
CV-9 Shuifen
CV-8 Shenque
CV-7 Yinjiao
CV-6 Qihai
CV-5 Shimen
CV-4 Guanyuan
CV-3 Zhongji
CV-2 Qugu

ST-15 Wuyi
ST-16 Yingchuang
ST-17 Ruzhong
ST-18 Rugen
ST-19 Burong
ST-20 Chengman
ST-21 Liangmen
ST-22 Guanmen
ST-23 Taiyi
ST-24 Huaroumen
ST-25 Tianshu
ST-26 Wailing
ST-27 Daju
ST-28 Shuidao
ST-29 Guilai
ST-30 Qichong

Stomach channel of foot-Yangming

Fig.1-1 (1) Anterior aspect acupuncture points, anatomical posture

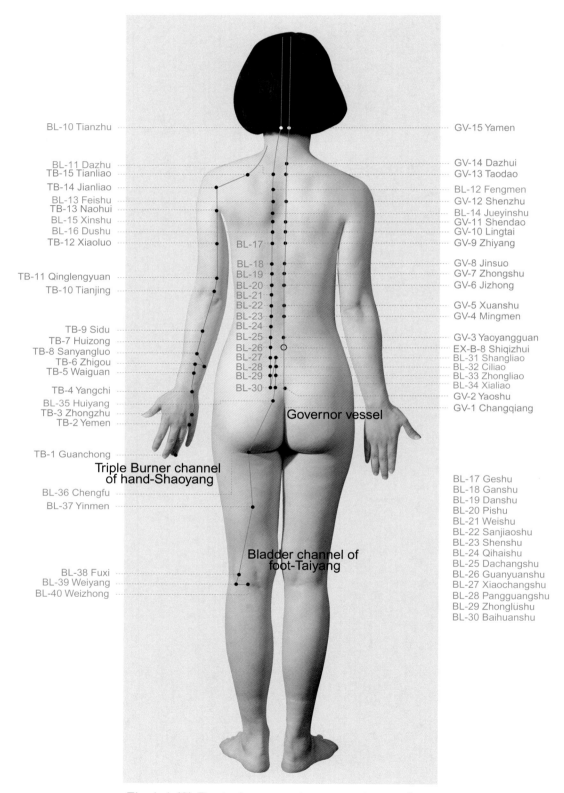

BL-10 Tianzhu
GV-15 Yamen

BL-11 Dazhu
TB-15 Tianliao
GV-14 Dazhui
GV-13 Taodao

TB-14 Jianliao
BL-12 Fengmen

BL-13 Feishu
TB-13 Naohui
GV-12 Shenzhu
BL-14 Jueyinshu

BL-15 Xinshu
GV-11 Shendao

BL-16 Dushu
GV-10 Lingtai

TB-12 Xiaoluo
GV-9 Zhiyang

BL-17

BL-18
GV-8 Jinsuo

BL-19
GV-7 Zhongshu

TB-11 Qinglengyuan
BL-20
GV-6 Jizhong

TB-10 Tianjing
BL-21

BL-22
GV-5 Xuanshu

BL-23
GV-4 Mingmen

BL-24

TB-9 Sidu
BL-25
GV-3 Yaoyangguan

TB-7 Huizong
BL-26
EX-B-8 Shiqizhui

TB-8 Sanyangluo
BL-27
BL-31 Shangliao

TB-6 Zhigou
BL-28
BL-32 Ciliao

TB-5 Waiguan
BL-29
BL-33 Zhongliao

BL-30
BL-34 Xialiao

TB-4 Yangchi
GV-2 Yaoshu

BL-35 Huiyang
GV-1 Changqiang

TB-3 Zhongzhu

TB-2 Yemen

TB-1 Guanchong

Governor vessel

**Triple Burner channel
of hand-Shaoyang**

BL-36 Chengfu
BL-17 Geshu
BL-18 Ganshu

BL-37 Yinmen
BL-19 Danshu
BL-20 Pishu
BL-21 Weishu
BL-22 Sanjiaoshu
BL-23 Shenshu
BL-24 Qihaishu
BL-25 Dachangshu
BL-26 Guanyuanshu
BL-27 Xiaochangshu
BL-28 Pangguangshu
BL-29 Zhonglüshu
BL-30 Baihuanshu

**Bladder channel of
foot-Taiyang**

BL-38 Fuxi
BL-39 Weiyang
BL-40 Weizhong

Fig.1-1 (2) Posterior aspect acupuncture points,
anatomical posture

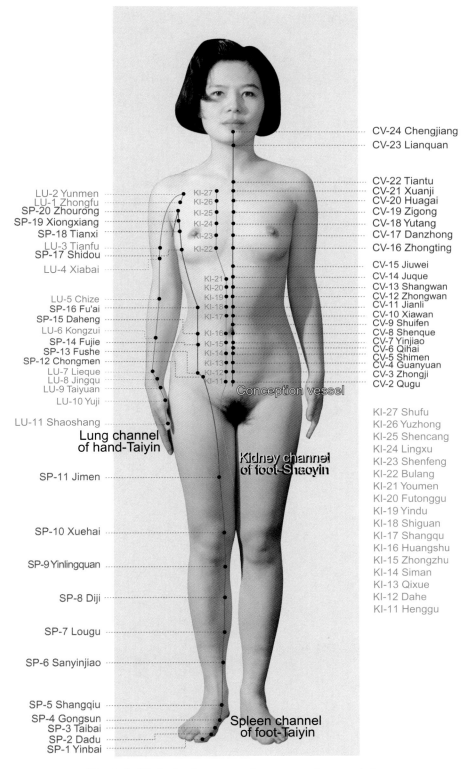

Fig.1-1 (3) Anterior aspect acupuncture points,
standing posture

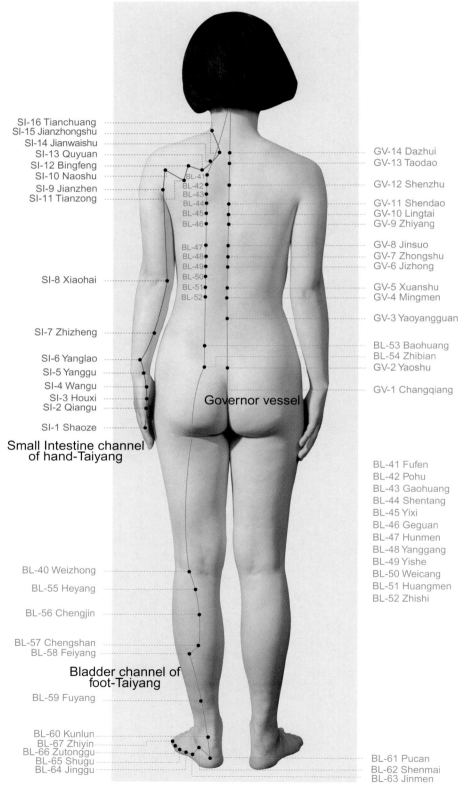

SI-16 Tianchuang
SI-15 Jianzhongshu
SI-14 Jianwaishu
SI-13 Quyuan
SI-12 Bingfeng
SI-10 Naoshu
SI-9 Jianzhen
SI-11 Tianzong

BL-41
BL-42
BL-43
BL-44
BL-45
BL-46

BL-47
BL-48
BL-49
BL-50
BL-51
BL-52

SI-8 Xiaohai

SI-7 Zhizheng

SI-6 Yanglao
SI-5 Yanggu
SI-4 Wangu
SI-3 Houxi
SI-2 Qiangu

SI-1 Shaoze

**Small Intestine channel
of hand-Taiyang**

Governor vessel

GV-14 Dazhui
GV-13 Taodao

GV-12 Shenzhu

GV-11 Shendao
GV-10 Lingtai
GV-9 Zhiyang

GV-8 Jinsuo
GV-7 Zhongshu
GV-6 Jizhong

GV-5 Xuanshu
GV-4 Mingmen

GV-3 Yaoyangguan

BL-53 Baohuang
BL-54 Zhibian
GV-2 Yaoshu

GV-1 Changqiang

BL-41 Fufen
BL-42 Pohu
BL-43 Gaohuang
BL-44 Shentang
BL-45 Yixi
BL-46 Geguan
BL-47 Hunmen
BL-48 Yanggang
BL-49 Yishe
BL-50 Weicang
BL-51 Huangmen
BL-52 Zhishi

BL-40 Weizhong

BL-55 Heyang

BL-56 Chengjin

BL-57 Chengshan
BL-58 Feiyang

**Bladder channel of
foot-Taiyang**

BL-59 Fuyang

BL-60 Kunlun
BL-67 Zhiyin
BL-66 Zutonggu
BL-65 Shugu
BL-64 Jinggu

BL-61 Pucan
BL-62 Shenmai
BL-63 Jinmen

Fig.1-1 (4) Posterior aspect acupuncture points,
standing posture

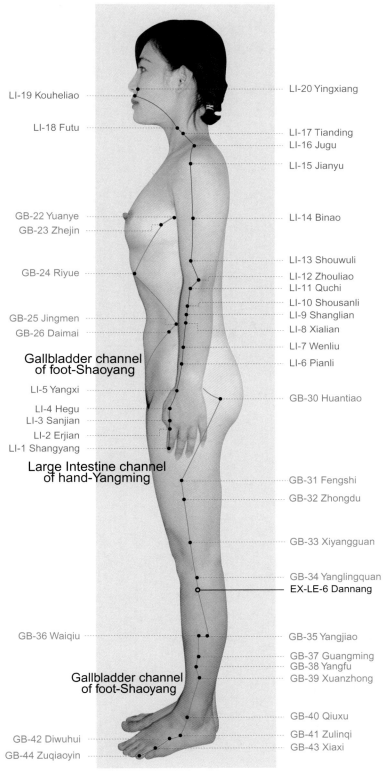

LI-19 Kouheliao

LI-18 Futu

GB-22 Yuanye
GB-23 Zhejin

GB-24 Riyue

GB-25 Jingmen
GB-26 Daimai

**Gallbladder channel
of foot-Shaoyang**

LI-5 Yangxi

LI-4 Hegu
LI-3 Sanjian

LI-2 Erjian
LI-1 Shangyang

**Large Intestine channel
of hand-Yangming**

GB-36 Waiqiu

**Gallbladder channel
of foot-Shaoyang**

GB-42 Diwuhui

GB-44 Zuqiaoyin

LI-20 Yingxiang

LI-17 Tianding
LI-16 Jugu

LI-15 Jianyu

LI-14 Binao

LI-13 Shouwuli
LI-12 Zhouliao
LI-11 Quchi
LI-10 Shousanli
LI-9 Shanglian
LI-8 Xialian
LI-7 Wenliu
LI-6 Pianli

GB-30 Huantiao

GB-31 Fengshi
GB-32 Zhongdu

GB-33 Xiyangguan

GB-34 Yanglingquan
EX-LE-6 Dannang

GB-35 Yangjiao

GB-37 Guangming
GB-38 Yangfu
GB-39 Xuanzhong

GB-40 Qiuxu

GB-41 Zulinqi
GB-43 Xiaxi

Fig.1-1 (5) Left lateral aspect acupuncture points,
standing posture

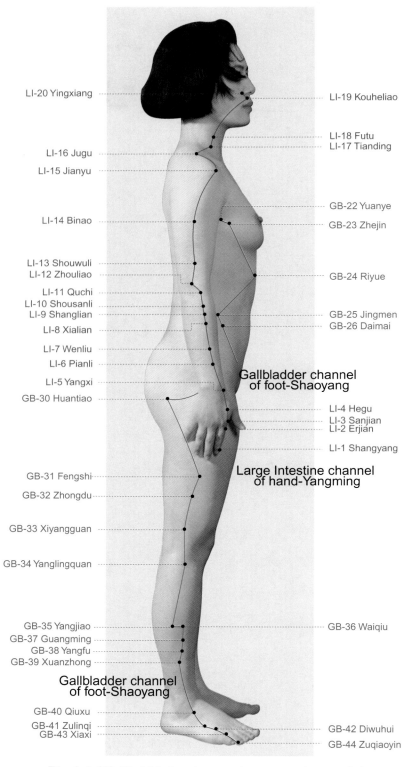

LI-20 Yingxiang
LI-16 Jugu
LI-15 Jianyu
LI-14 Binao
LI-13 Shouwuli
LI-12 Zhouliao
LI-11 Quchi
LI-10 Shousanli
LI-9 Shanglian
LI-8 Xialian
LI-7 Wenliu
LI-6 Pianli
LI-5 Yangxi
GB-30 Huantiao
GB-31 Fengshi
GB-32 Zhongdu
GB-33 Xiyangguan
GB-34 Yanglingquan
GB-35 Yangjiao
GB-37 Guangming
GB-38 Yangfu
GB-39 Xuanzhong
GB-40 Qiuxu
GB-41 Zulinqi
GB-43 Xiaxi

LI-19 Kouheliao
LI-18 Futu
LI-17 Tianding
GB-22 Yuanye
GB-23 Zhejin
GB-24 Riyue
GB-25 Jingmen
GB-26 Daimai

**Gallbladder channel
of foot-Shaoyang**

LI-4 Hegu
LI-3 Sanjian
LI-2 Erjian
LI-1 Shangyang

**Large Intestine channel
of hand-Yangming**

GB-36 Waiqiu

**Gallbladder channel
of foot-Shaoyang**

GB-42 Diwuhui
GB-44 Zuqiaoyin

Fig.1-1 (6) Right lateral aspect acupuncture points,
standing posture

FIGURES OF ACUPUNCTURE POINTS, CASUAL POSTURE

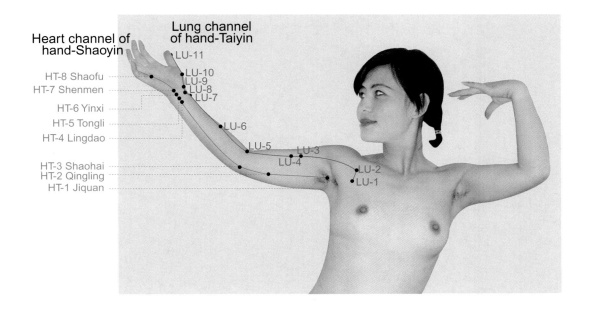

Heart channel of hand-Shaoyin

Lung channel of hand-Taiyin

LU-11

LU-10
LU-9
LU-8
LU-7

HT-8 Shaofu
HT-7 Shenmen
HT-6 Yinxi
HT-5 Tongli
HT-4 Lingdao

LU-6

LU-5
LU-3
LU-4

HT-3 Shaohai
HT-2 Qingling
HT-1 Jiquan

LU-2
LU-1

LU-1 Zhongfu
LU-2 Yunmen
LU-3 Tianfu
LU-4 Xiabai

LU-5 Chize
LU-6 Kongzui
LU-7 Lieque
LU-8 Jingqu

LU-9 Taiyuan
LU-10 Yuji
LU-11 Shaoshang

Fig.1-2 (1) Points on the Lung and Heart channels

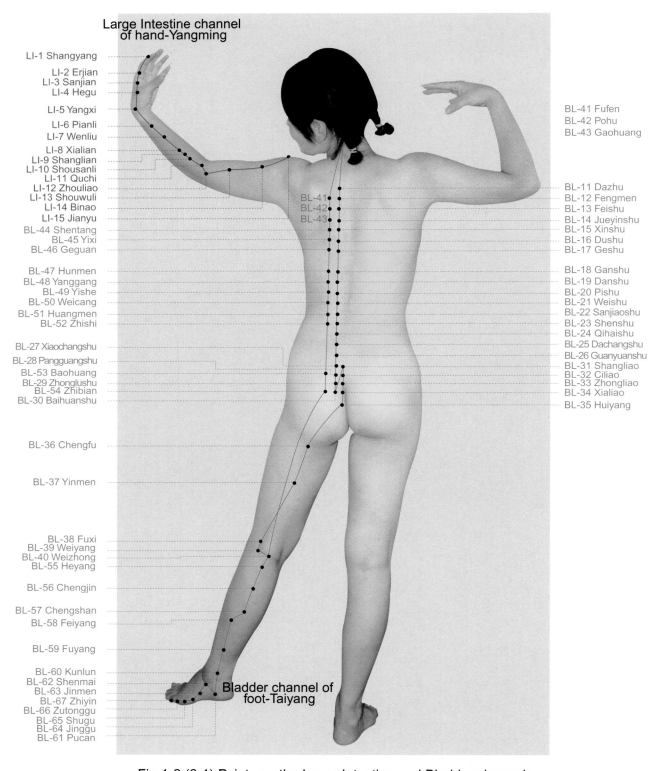

Large Intestine channel of hand-Yangming

LI-1 Shangyang
LI-2 Erjian
LI-3 Sanjian
LI-4 Hegu
LI-5 Yangxi
LI-6 Pianli
LI-7 Wenliu
LI-8 Xialian
LI-9 Shanglian
LI-10 Shousanli
LI-11 Quchi
LI-12 Zhouliao
LI-13 Shouwuli
LI-14 Binao
LI-15 Jianyu
BL-44 Shentang
BL-45 Yixi
BL-46 Geguan
BL-47 Hunmen
BL-48 Yanggang
BL-49 Yishe
BL-50 Weicang
BL-51 Huangmen
BL-52 Zhishi
BL-27 Xiaochangshu
BL-28 Pangguangshu
BL-53 Baohuang
BL-29 Zhonglüshu
BL-54 Zhibian
BL-30 Baihuanshu
BL-36 Chengfu
BL-37 Yinmen
BL-38 Fuxi
BL-39 Weiyang
BL-40 Weizhong
BL-55 Heyang
BL-56 Chengjin
BL-57 Chengshan
BL-58 Feiyang
BL-59 Fuyang
BL-60 Kunlun
BL-62 Shenmai
BL-63 Jinmen
BL-67 Zhiyin
BL-66 Zutonggu
BL-65 Shugu
BL-64 Jinggu
BL-61 Pucan

BL-41 Fufen
BL-42 Pohu
BL-43 Gaohuang
BL-11 Dazhu
BL-12 Fengmen
BL-13 Feishu
BL-14 Jueyinshu
BL-15 Xinshu
BL-16 Dushu
BL-17 Geshu
BL-18 Ganshu
BL-19 Danshu
BL-20 Pishu
BL-21 Weishu
BL-22 Sanjiaoshu
BL-23 Shenshu
BL-24 Qihaishu
BL-25 Dachangshu
BL-26 Guanyuanshu
BL-31 Shangliao
BL-32 Ciliao
BL-33 Zhongliao
BL-34 Xialiao
BL-35 Huiyang

BL-41
BL-42
BL-43

Bladder channel of foot-Taiyang

Fig.1-2 (2-1) Points on the Large Intestine and Bladder channels

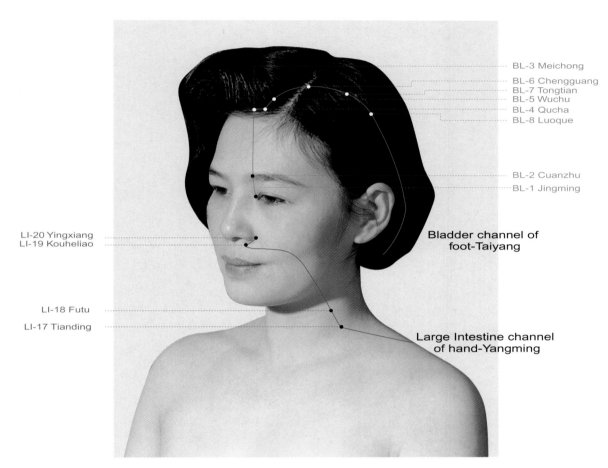

BL-3 Meichong
BL-6 Chengguang
BL-7 Tongtian
BL-5 Wuchu
BL-4 Qucha
BL-8 Luoque

BL-2 Cuanzhu
BL-1 Jingming

Bladder channel of foot-Taiyang

LI-20 Yingxiang
LI-19 Kouheliao

LI-18 Futu

LI-17 Tianding

Large Intestine channel of hand-Yangming

Fig.1-2 (2-2) Large Intestine and Bladder channel points
on the head and neck

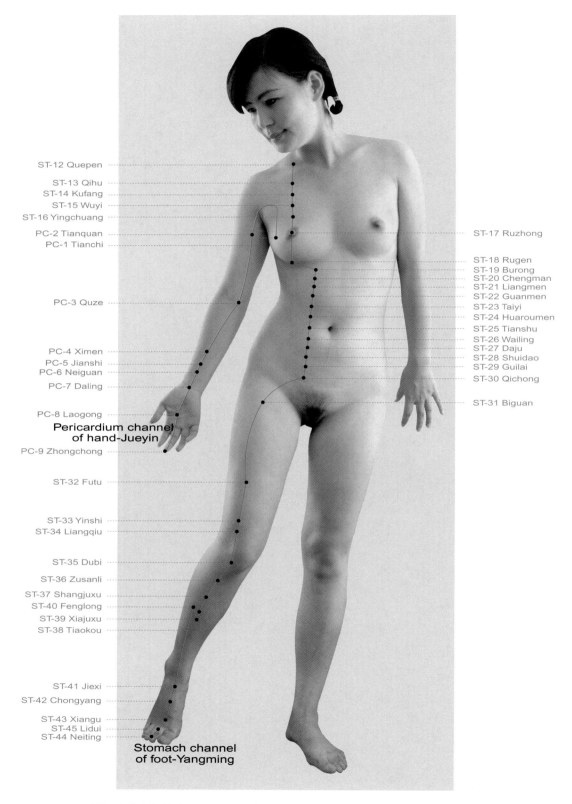

ST-12 Quepen

ST-13 Qihu
ST-14 Kufang
ST-15 Wuyi
ST-16 Yingchuang

PC-2 Tianquan
PC-1 Tianchi

PC-3 Quze

PC-4 Ximen
PC-5 Jianshi
PC-6 Neiguan

PC-7 Daling

PC-8 Laogong

**Pericardium channel
of hand-Jueyin**

PC-9 Zhongchong

ST-32 Futu

ST-33 Yinshi
ST-34 Liangqiu

ST-35 Dubi

ST-36 Zusanli

ST-37 Shangjuxu
ST-40 Fenglong
ST-39 Xiajuxu
ST-38 Tiaokou

ST-41 Jiexi
ST-42 Chongyang

ST-43 Xiangu
ST-45 Lidui
ST-44 Neiting

ST-17 Ruzhong

ST-18 Rugen
ST-19 Burong
ST-20 Chengman
ST-21 Liangmen
ST-22 Guanmen
ST-23 Taiyi
ST-24 Huaroumen
ST-25 Tianshu
ST-26 Wailing
ST-27 Daju
ST-28 Shuidao
ST-29 Guilai
ST-30 Qichong

ST-31 Biguan

**Stomach channel
of foot-Yangming**

Fig.1-2 (3) Points on the Stomach and Pericardium channels

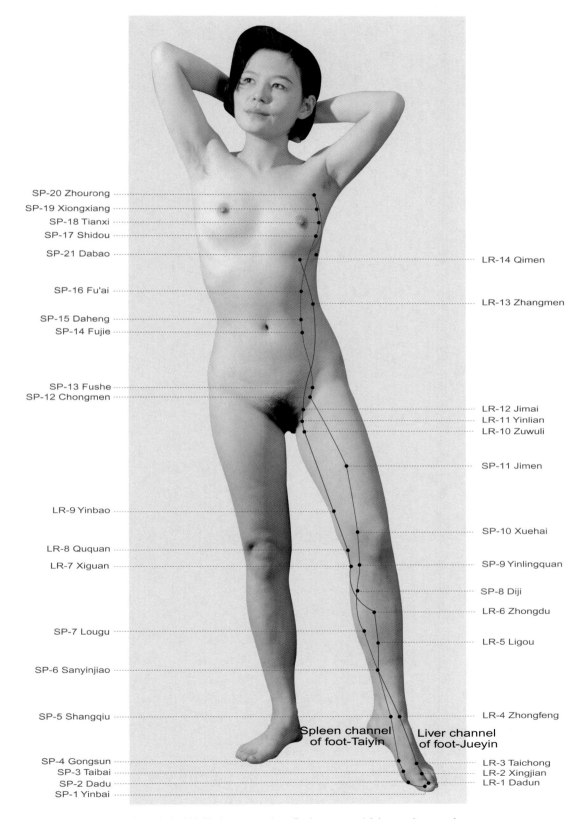

SP-20 Zhourong
SP-19 Xiongxiang
SP-18 Tianxi
SP-17 Shidou
SP-21 Dabao
SP-16 Fu'ai
SP-15 Daheng
SP-14 Fujie
SP-13 Fushe
SP-12 Chongmen
LR-9 Yinbao
LR-8 Ququan
LR-7 Xiguan
SP-7 Lougu
SP-6 Sanyinjiao
SP-5 Shangqiu
SP-4 Gongsun
SP-3 Taibai
SP-2 Dadu
SP-1 Yinbai

LR-14 Qimen
LR-13 Zhangmen
LR-12 Jimai
LR-11 Yinlian
LR-10 Zuwuli
SP-11 Jimen
SP-10 Xuehai
SP-9 Yinlingquan
SP-8 Diji
LR-6 Zhongdu
LR-5 Ligou
LR-4 Zhongfeng
LR-3 Taichong
LR-2 Xingjian
LR-1 Dadun

Spleen channel
of foot-Taiyin

Liver channel
of foot-Jueyin

Fig.1-2 (4) Points on the Spleen and Liver channels

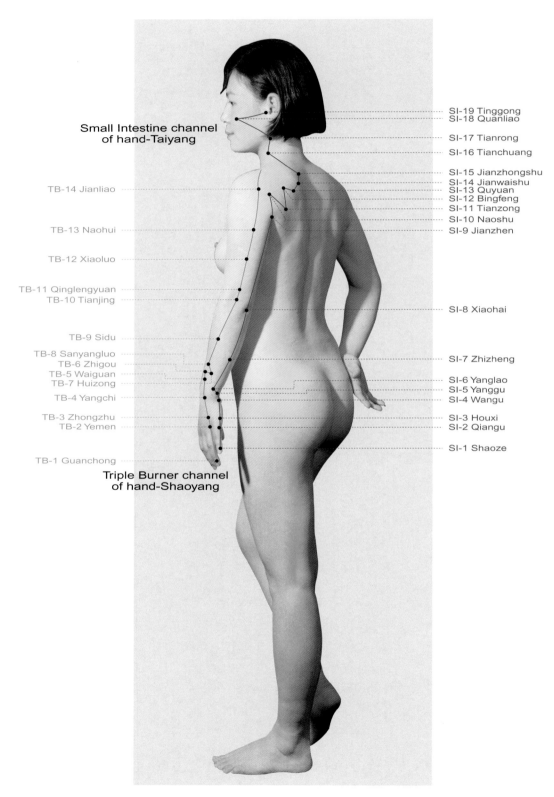

Small Intestine channel
of hand-Taiyang

SI-19 Tinggong
SI-18 Quanliao
SI-17 Tianrong
SI-16 Tianchuang
SI-15 Jianzhongshu
SI-14 Jianwaishu
SI-13 Quyuan
SI-12 Bingfeng
SI-11 Tianzong
SI-10 Naoshu
SI-9 Jianzhen

TB-14 Jianliao

TB-13 Naohui

TB-12 Xiaoluo

TB-11 Qinglengyuan
TB-10 Tianjing

SI-8 Xiaohai

TB-9 Sidu
TB-8 Sanyangluo
TB-6 Zhigou
TB-5 Waiguan
TB-7 Huizong
TB-4 Yangchi

SI-7 Zhizheng
SI-6 Yanglao
SI-5 Yanggu
SI-4 Wangu

TB-3 Zhongzhu
TB-2 Yemen

SI-3 Houxi
SI-2 Qiangu
SI-1 Shaoze

TB-1 Guanchong
Triple Burner channel
of hand-Shaoyang

Fig.1-2 (5) Points on the Small Intestine and Triple Burner channels

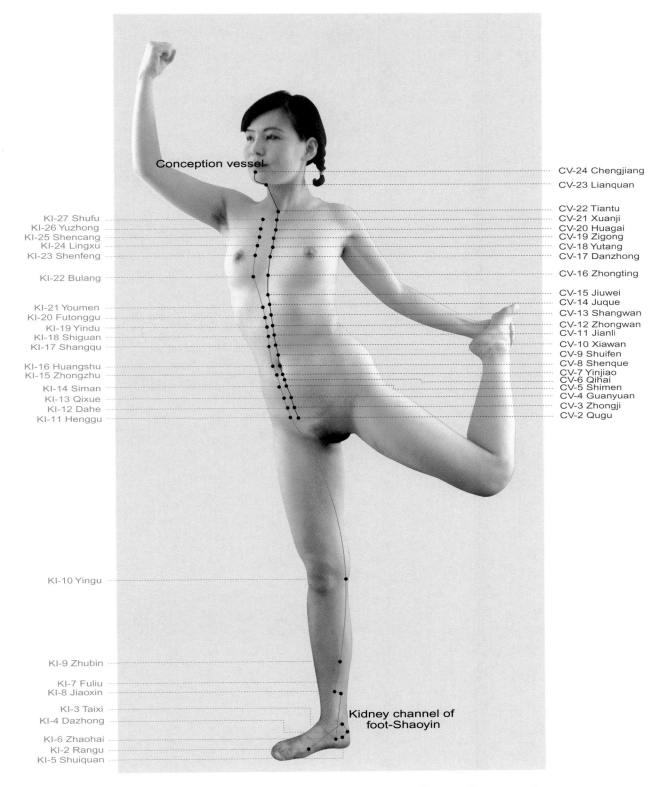

Conception vessel

KI-27 Shufu
KI-26 Yuzhong
KI-25 Shencang
KI-24 Lingxu
KI-23 Shenfeng

KI-22 Bulang

KI-21 Youmen
KI-20 Futonggu
KI-19 Yindu
KI-18 Shiguan
KI-17 Shangqu

KI-16 Huangshu
KI-15 Zhongzhu
KI-14 Siman
KI-13 Qixue
KI-12 Dahe
KI-11 Henggu

KI-10 Yingu

KI-9 Zhubin

KI-7 Fuliu
KI-8 Jiaoxin

KI-3 Taixi
KI-4 Dazhong

KI-6 Zhaohai
KI-2 Rangu
KI-5 Shuiquan

CV-24 Chengjiang
CV-23 Lianquan

CV-22 Tiantu
CV-21 Xuanji
CV-20 Huagai
CV-19 Zigong
CV-18 Yutang
CV-17 Danzhong

CV-16 Zhongting

CV-15 Jiuwei
CV-14 Juque
CV-13 Shangwan
CV-12 Zhongwan
CV-11 Jianli
CV-10 Xiawan
CV-9 Shuifen
CV-8 Shenque
CV-7 Yinjiao
CV-6 Qihai
CV-5 Shimen
CV-4 Guanyuan
CV-3 Zhongji
CV-2 Qugu

Kidney channel of
foot-Shaoyin

Fig.1-2(6) Points on the Kidney channel and Conception vessel

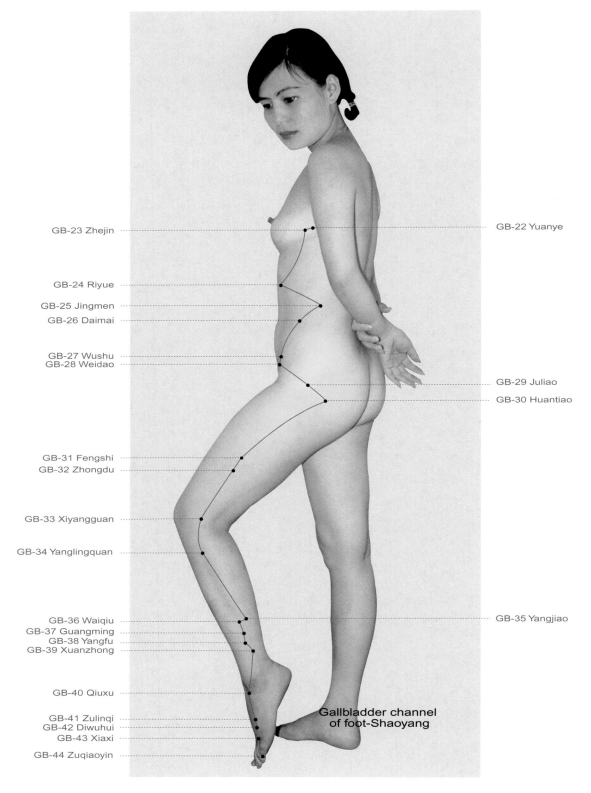

GB-23 Zhejin
GB-22 Yuanye

GB-24 Riyue

GB-25 Jingmen
GB-26 Daimai

GB-27 Wushu
GB-28 Weidao

GB-29 Juliao
GB-30 Huantiao

GB-31 Fengshi
GB-32 Zhongdu

GB-33 Xiyangguan

GB-34 Yanglingquan

GB-36 Waiqiu
GB-37 Guangming
GB-38 Yangfu
GB-39 Xuanzhong

GB-35 Yangjiao

GB-40 Qiuxu

GB-41 Zulinqi
GB-42 Diwuhui
GB-43 Xiaxi

GB-44 Zuqiaoyin

Gallbladder channel
of foot-Shaoyang

Fig.1-2 (7-1) Points on the Gallbladder channel

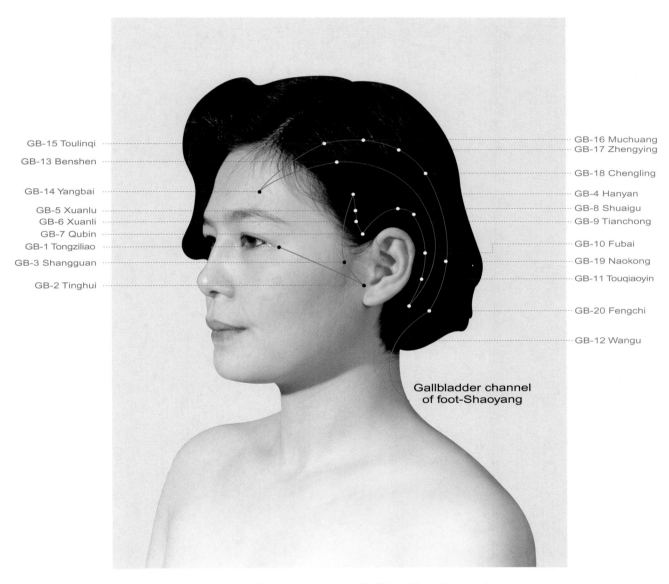

GB-15 Toulinqi
GB-13 Benshen
GB-14 Yangbai
GB-5 Xuanlu
GB-6 Xuanli
GB-7 Qubin
GB-1 Tongziliao
GB-3 Shangguan
GB-2 Tinghui

GB-16 Muchuang
GB-17 Zhengying
GB-18 Chengling
GB-4 Hanyan
GB-8 Shuaigu
GB-9 Tianchong
GB-10 Fubai
GB-19 Naokong
GB-11 Touqiaoyin
GB-20 Fengchi
GB-12 Wangu

Gallbladder channel
of foot-Shaoyang

Fig.1-2 (7-2) Points on the Gallbladder channel
(lateral aspect of the head and neck)

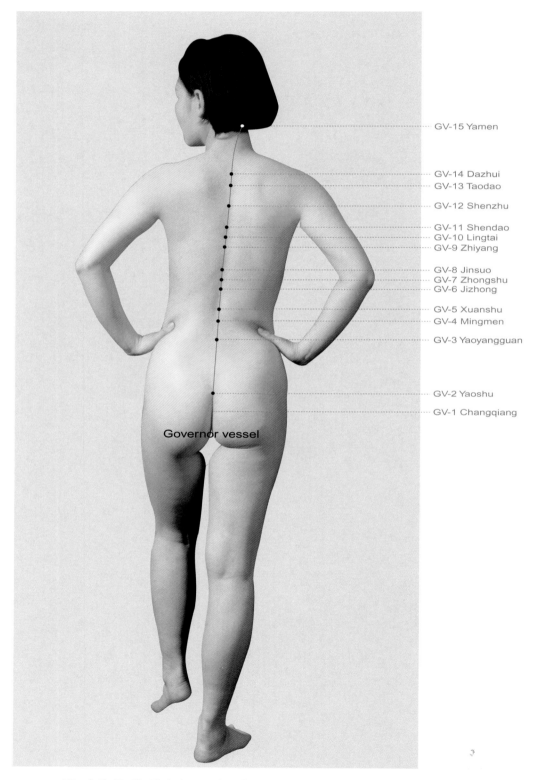

GV-15 Yamen

GV-14 Dazhui
GV-13 Taodao

GV-12 Shenzhu

GV-11 Shendao
GV-10 Lingtai
GV-9 Zhiyang

GV-8 Jinsuo
GV-7 Zhongshu
GV-6 Jizhong

GV-5 Xuanshu
GV-4 Mingmen

GV-3 Yaoyangguan

GV-2 Yaoshu

GV-1 Changqiang

Governor vessel

Fig.1-2 (8-1) Points on the Governor vessel

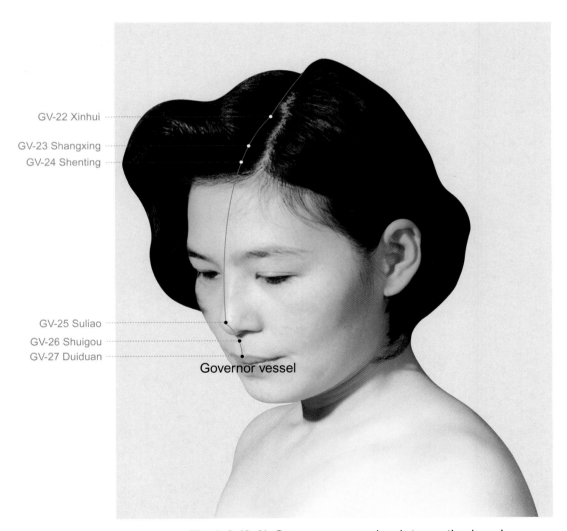

GV-22 Xinhui

GV-23 Shangxing

GV-24 Shenting

GV-25 Suliao

GV-26 Shuigou

GV-27 Duiduan

Governor vessel

Fig.1-2 (8-2) Governor vessel points on the head

2 Regional figures of acupuncture points

FIGURES OF ACUPUNCTURE POINTS ON THE TRUNK

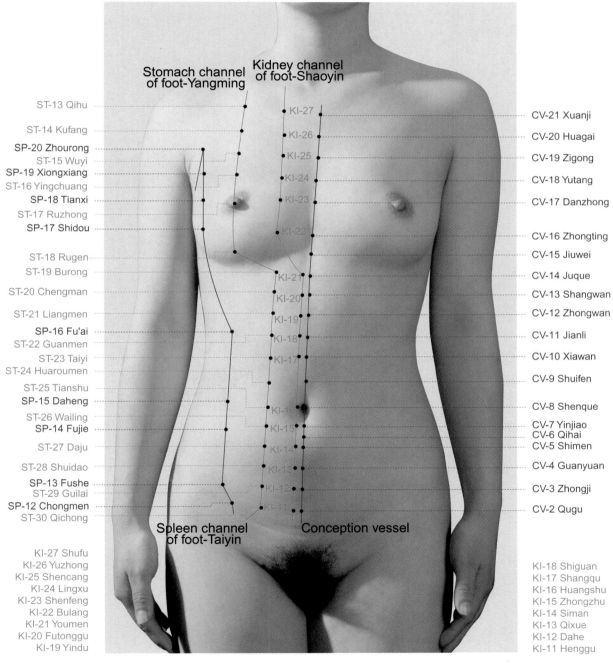

Fig.2-1 (1) Acupuncture points, anterior aspect of the trunk

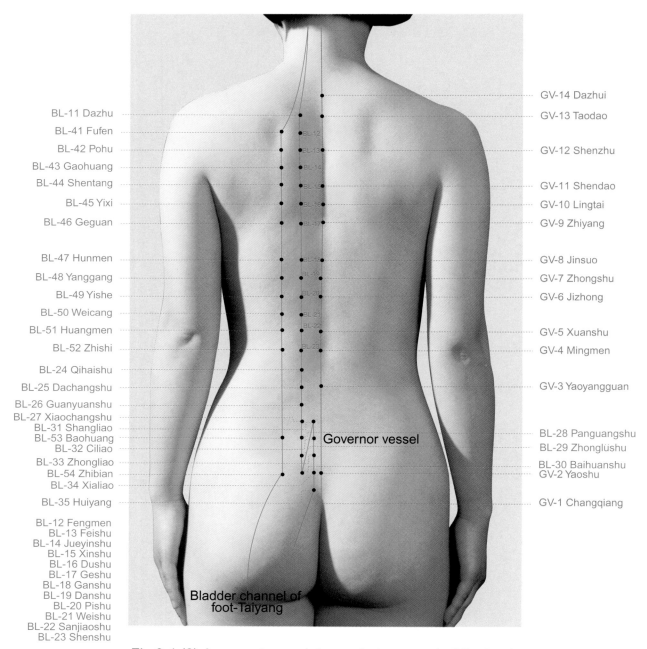

BL-11 Dazhu
BL-41 Fufen
BL-42 Pohu
BL-43 Gaohuang
BL-44 Shentang
BL-45 Yixi
BL-46 Geguan

BL-47 Hunmen
BL-48 Yanggang
BL-49 Yishe
BL-50 Weicang
BL-51 Huangmen
BL-52 Zhishi

BL-24 Qihaishu
BL-25 Dachangshu
BL-26 Guanyuanshu
BL-27 Xiaochangshu
BL-31 Shangliao
BL-53 Baohuang
BL-32 Ciliao
BL-33 Zhongliao
BL-54 Zhibian
BL-34 Xialiao
BL-35 Huiyang

BL-12 Fengmen
BL-13 Feishu
BL-14 Jueyinshu
BL-15 Xinshu
BL-16 Dushu
BL-17 Geshu
BL-18 Ganshu
BL-19 Danshu
BL-20 Pishu
BL-21 Weishu
BL-22 Sanjiaoshu
BL-23 Shenshu

GV-14 Dazhui
GV-13 Taodao
GV-12 Shenzhu
GV-11 Shendao
GV-10 Lingtai
GV-9 Zhiyang
GV-8 Jinsuo
GV-7 Zhongshu
GV-6 Jizhong
GV-5 Xuanshu
GV-4 Mingmen
GV-3 Yaoyangguan
BL-28 Panguangshu
BL-29 Zhonglüshu
BL-30 Baihuanshu
GV-2 Yaoshu
GV-1 Changqiang

Governor vessel

Bladder channel of foot-Taiyang

Fig.2-1 (2) Acupuncture points, posterior aspect of the trunk

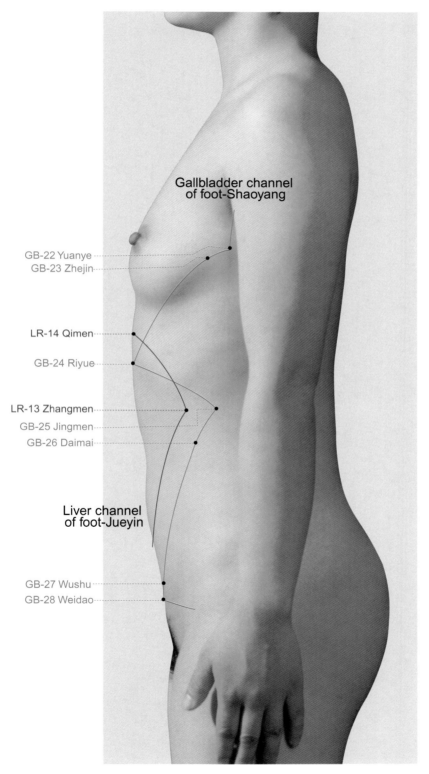

Fig.2-1 (3) Acupuncture points, left lateral aspect of the trunk

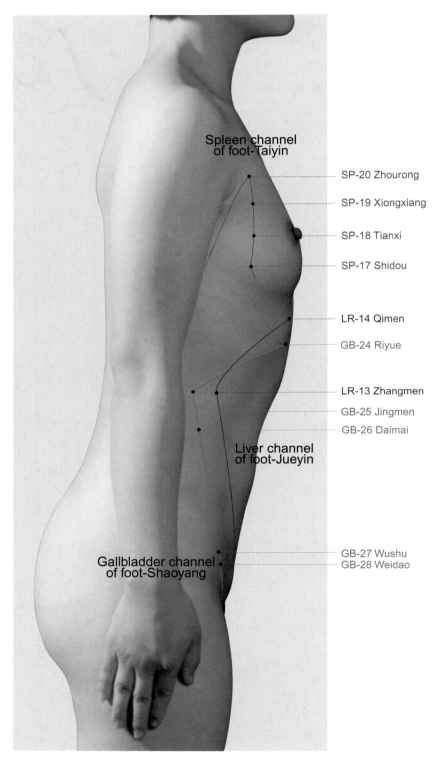

Spleen channel
of foot-Taiyin

SP-20 Zhourong

SP-19 Xiongxiang

SP-18 Tianxi

SP-17 Shidou

LR-14 Qimen

GB-24 Riyue

LR-13 Zhangmen

GB-25 Jingmen

GB-26 Daimai

Liver channel
of foot-Jueyin

Gallbladder channel
of foot-Shaoyang

GB-27 Wushu
GB-28 Weidao

Fig.2-1 (4) Acupuncture points, right lateral aspect of the trunk

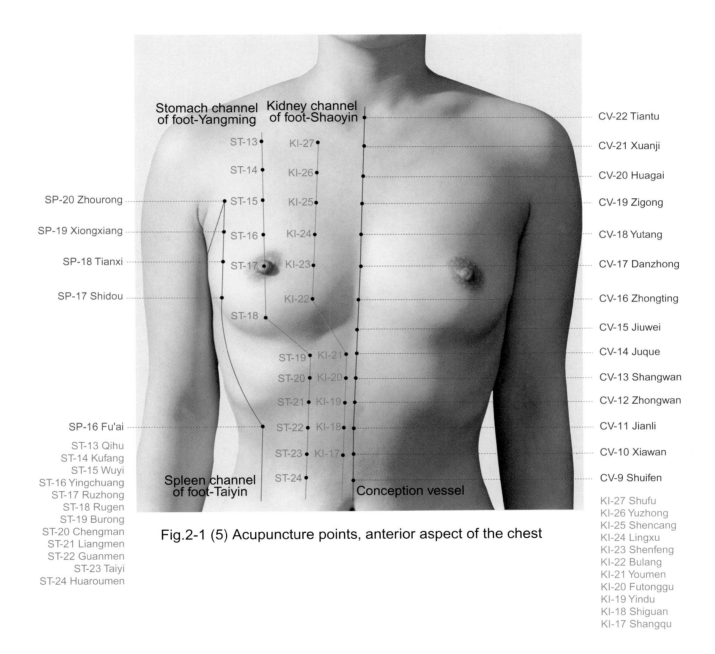

Stomach channel
of foot-Yangming

Kidney channel
of foot-Shaoyin

CV-22 Tiantu
CV-21 Xuanji
CV-20 Huagai
CV-19 Zigong
CV-18 Yutang
CV-17 Danzhong
CV-16 Zhongting
CV-15 Jiuwei
CV-14 Juque
CV-13 Shangwan
CV-12 Zhongwan
CV-11 Jianli
CV-10 Xiawan
CV-9 Shuifen

ST-13
ST-14
ST-15
ST-16
ST-17
ST-18
ST-19
ST-20
ST-21
ST-22
ST-23
ST-24

KI-27
KI-26
KI-25
KI-24
KI-23
KI-22
KI-21
KI-20
KI-19
KI-18
KI-17

SP-20 Zhourong
SP-19 Xiongxiang
SP-18 Tianxi
SP-17 Shidou
SP-16 Fu'ai

ST-13 Qihu
ST-14 Kufang
ST-15 Wuyi
ST-16 Yingchuang
ST-17 Ruzhong
ST-18 Rugen
ST-19 Burong
ST-20 Chengman
ST-21 Liangmen
ST-22 Guanmen
ST-23 Taiyi
ST-24 Huaroumen

Spleen channel
of foot-Taiyin

Conception vessel

KI-27 Shufu
KI-26 Yuzhong
KI-25 Shencang
KI-24 Lingxu
KI-23 Shenfeng
KI-22 Bulang
KI-21 Youmen
KI-20 Futonggu
KI-19 Yindu
KI-18 Shiguan
KI-17 Shangqu

Fig.2-1 (5) Acupuncture points, anterior aspect of the chest

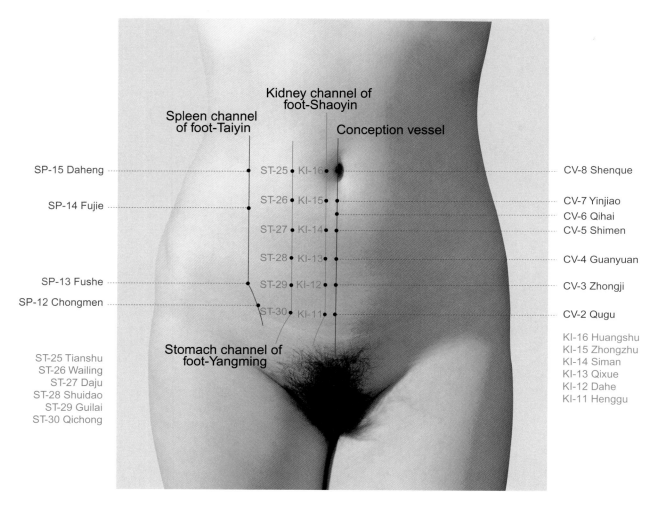

Kidney channel of
foot-Shaoyin

Spleen channel
of foot-Taiyin

Conception vessel

SP-15 Daheng ········· ST-25 ● KI-16 ●   ●········· CV-8 Shenque

SP-14 Fujie ········· ST-26 ● KI-15 ●   ●········· CV-7 Yinjiao
                                                ●········· CV-6 Qihai
                    ST-27 ● KI-14 ●   ●········· CV-5 Shimen

                    ST-28 ● KI-13 ●   ●········· CV-4 Guanyuan

SP-13 Fushe ········· ST-29 ● KI-12 ●   ●········· CV-3 Zhongji

SP-12 Chongmen ········· ST-30 ● KI-11 ●   ●········· CV-2 Qugu

Stomach channel of
foot-Yangming

ST-25 Tianshu
ST-26 Wailing
ST-27 Daju
ST-28 Shuidao
ST-29 Guilai
ST-30 Qichong

KI-16 Huangshu
KI-15 Zhongzhu
KI-14 Siman
KI-13 Qixue
KI-12 Dahe
KI-11 Henggu

Fig.2-1 (6) Acupuncture points on the abdomen

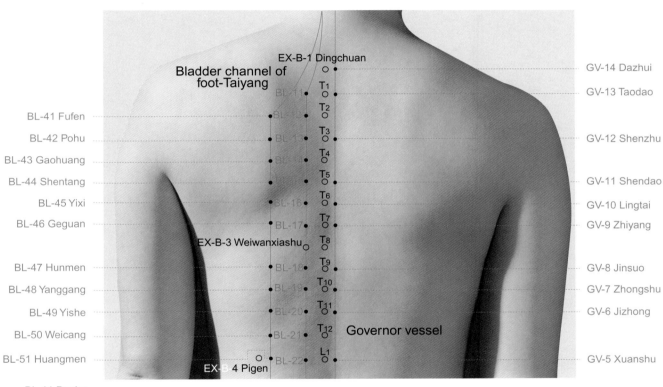

EX-B-1 Dingchuan

Bladder channel of
foot-Taiyang

GV-14 Dazhui

GV-13 Taodao

BL-41 Fufen

BL-42 Pohu

BL-43 Gaohuang

BL-44 Shentang

BL-45 Yixi

BL-46 Geguan

EX-B-3 Weiwanxiashu

BL-47 Hunmen

BL-48 Yanggang

BL-49 Yishe

BL-50 Weicang

BL-51 Huangmen

EX-B-4 Pigen

GV-12 Shenzhu

GV-11 Shendao

GV-10 Lingtai

GV-9 Zhiyang

GV-8 Jinsuo

GV-7 Zhongshu

GV-6 Jizhong

Governor vessel

GV-5 Xuanshu

T1
T2
T3
T4
T5
T6
T7
T8
T9
T10
T11
T12
L1

BL-11 Dazhu
BL-12 Fengmen
BL-13 Feishu
BL-14 Jueyinshu
BL-15 Xinshu
BL-16 Dushu
BL-17 Geshu
BL-18 Ganshu
BL-19 Danshu
BL-20 Pishu
BL-21 Weishu
BL-22 Sanjiaoshu

Fig.2-1 (7) Acupuncture points on the back

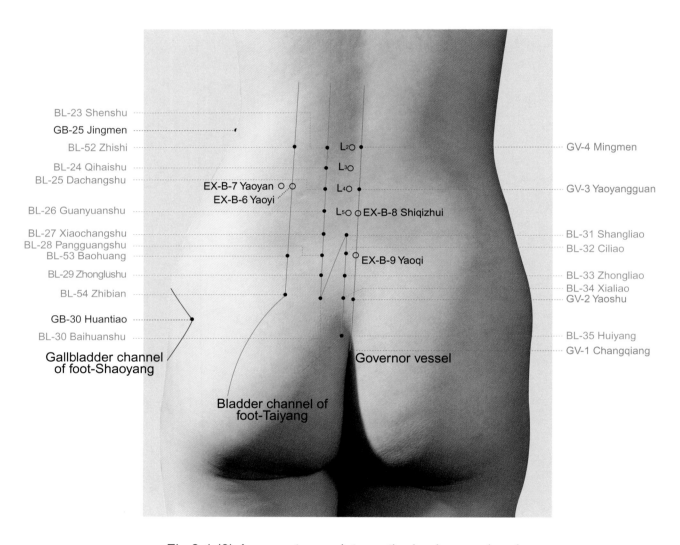

Fig.2-1 (8) Acupuncture points on the lumbosacral region

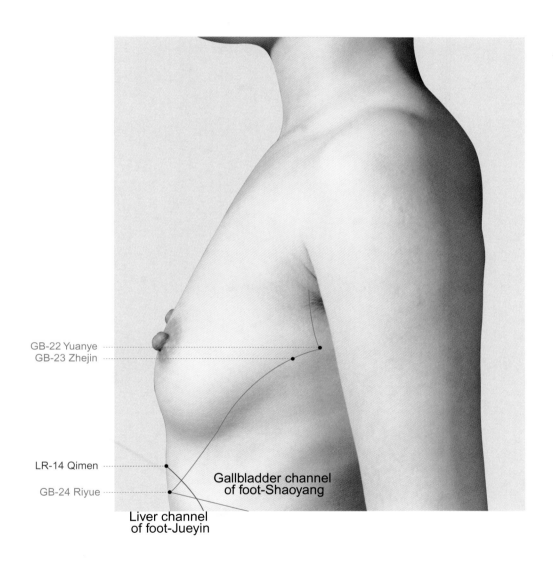

GB-22 Yuanye
GB-23 Zhejin

LR-14 Qimen

GB-24 Riyue

Gallbladder channel
of foot-Shaoyang

Liver channel
of foot-Jueyin

Fig.2-1 (9) Acupuncture points, lateral aspect of the chest

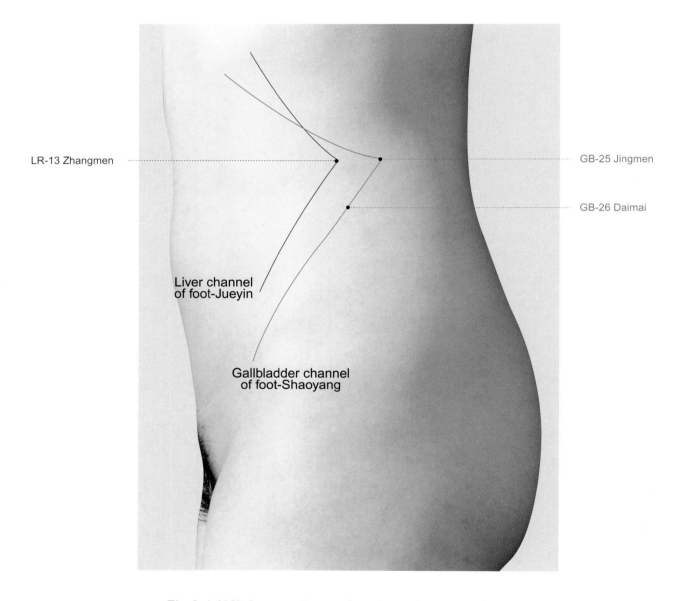

LR-13 Zhangmen

GB-25 Jingmen

GB-26 Daimai

Liver channel
of foot-Jueyin

Gallbladder channel
of foot-Shaoyang

Fig.2-1 (10) Acupuncture points, lateral aspect of the hip

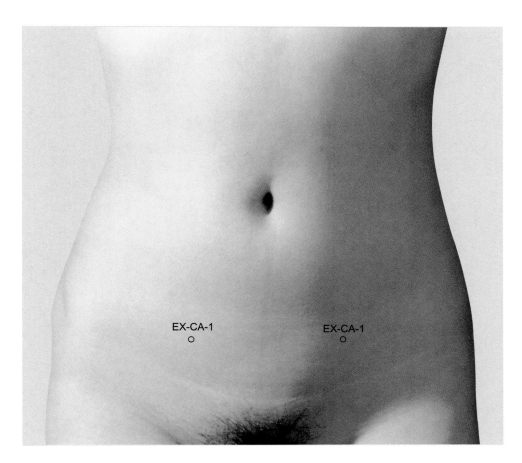

EX-CA-1 Zigong

Fig.2-1 (11) Extraordinary acupuncture points on the abdomen

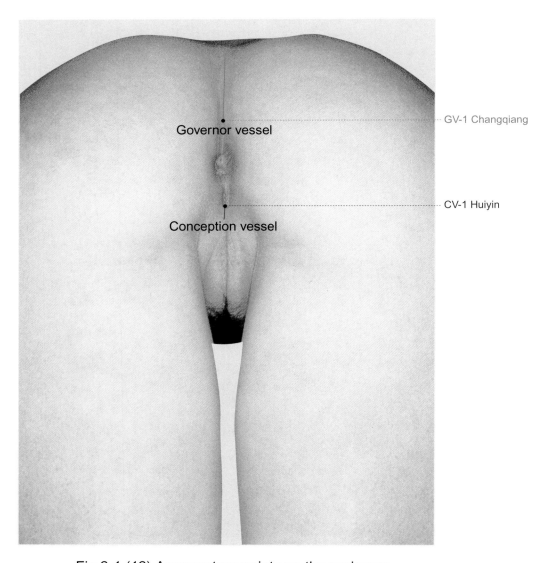

Fig.2-1 (12) Acupuncture points on the perineum

FIGURES OF ACUPUNCTURE POINTS ON THE HEAD AND NECK

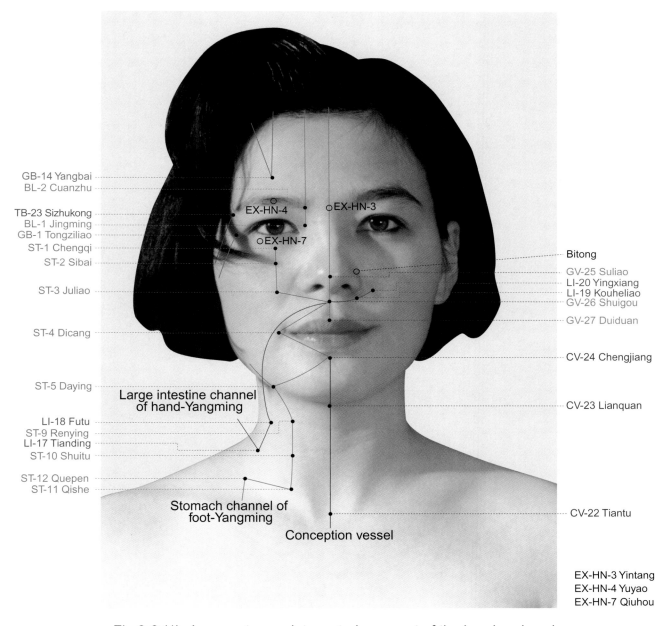

GB-14 Yangbai
BL-2 Cuanzhu

TB-23 Sizhukong
BL-1 Jingming
GB-1 Tongziliao
ST-1 Chengqi
ST-2 Sibai

ST-3 Juliao

ST-4 Dicang

ST-5 Daying

Large intestine channel
of hand-Yangming

LI-18 Futu
ST-9 Renying
LI-17 Tianding
ST-10 Shuitu

ST-12 Quepen
ST-11 Qishe

Stomach channel of
foot-Yangming

Conception vessel

EX-HN-4
EX-HN-3
EX-HN-7

Bitong
GV-25 Suliao
LI-20 Yingxiang
LI-19 Kouheliao
GV-26 Shuigou
GV-27 Duiduan

CV-24 Chengjiang

CV-23 Lianquan

CV-22 Tiantu

EX-HN-3 Yintang
EX-HN-4 Yuyao
EX-HN-7 Qiuhou

Fig.2-2 (1) Acupuncture points, anterior aspect of the head and neck

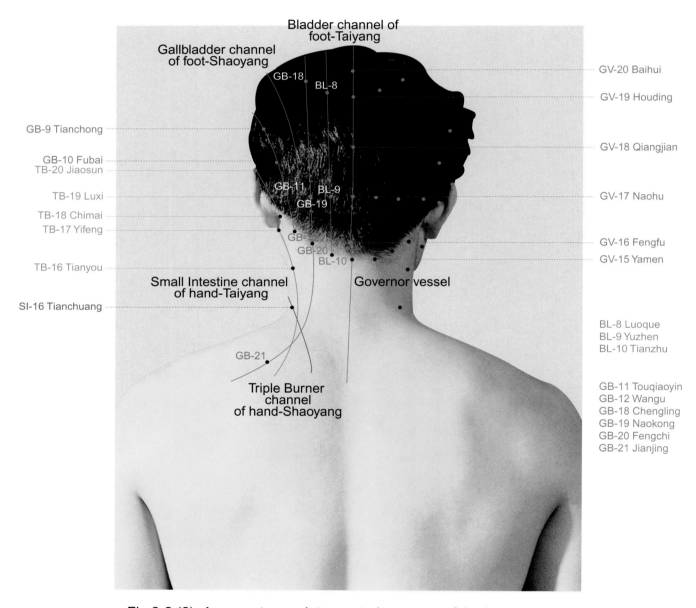

Bladder channel of foot-Taiyang

Gallbladder channel of foot-Shaoyang

GB-18

BL-8

GV-20 Baihui

GV-19 Houding

GB-9 Tianchong

GB-10 Fubai
TB-20 Jiaosun

GV-18 Qiangjian

TB-19 Luxi

GB-11 BL-9

GB-19

GV-17 Naohu

TB-18 Chimai

TB-17 Yifeng

GB-20

BL-10

GV-16 Fengfu

GV-15 Yamen

TB-16 Tianyou

Small Intestine channel of hand-Taiyang

Governor vessel

SI-16 Tianchuang

BL-8 Luoque
BL-9 Yuzhen
BL-10 Tianzhu

GB-21

Triple Burner channel of hand-Shaoyang

GB-11 Touqiaoyin
GB-12 Wangu
GB-18 Chengling
GB-19 Naokong
GB-20 Fengchi
GB-21 Jianjing

Fig.2-2 (2) Acupuncture points, posterior aspect of the head and neck

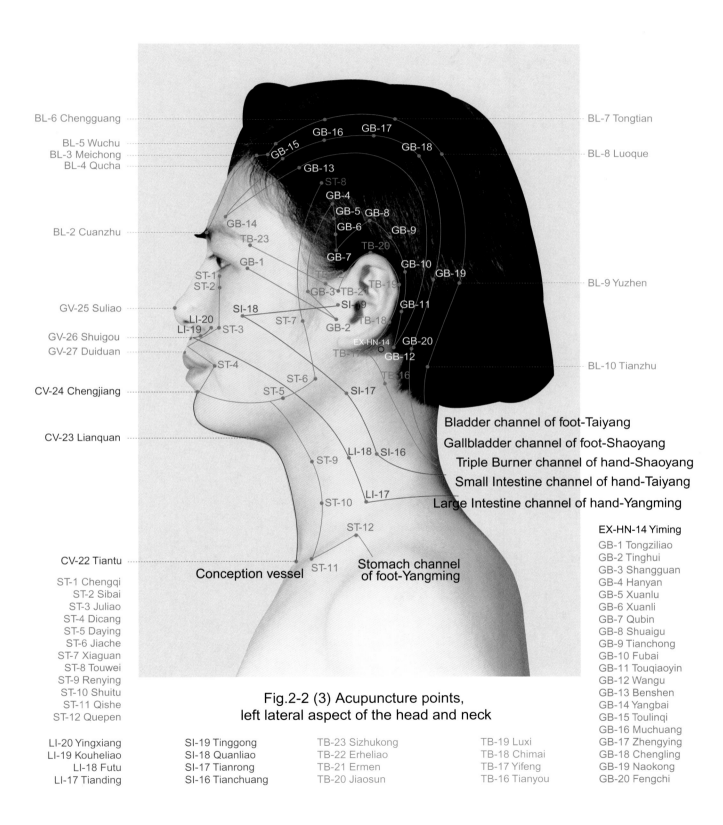

Fig.2-2 (3) Acupuncture points,
left lateral aspect of the head and neck

BL-6 Chengguang
BL-5 Wuchu
BL-3 Meichong
BL-4 Qucha
BL-2 Cuanzhu
GV-25 Suliao
GV-26 Shuigou
GV-27 Duiduan
CV-24 Chengjiang
CV-23 Lianquan
CV-22 Tiantu

BL-7 Tongtian
BL-8 Luoque
BL-9 Yuzhen
BL-10 Tianzhu

Bladder channel of foot-Taiyang
Gallbladder channel of foot-Shaoyang
Triple Burner channel of hand-Shaoyang
Small Intestine channel of hand-Taiyang
Large Intestine channel of hand-Yangming

Conception vessel

Stomach channel
of foot-Yangming

ST-1 Chengqi
ST-2 Sibai
ST-3 Juliao
ST-4 Dicang
ST-5 Daying
ST-6 Jiache
ST-7 Xiaguan
ST-8 Touwei
ST-9 Renying
ST-10 Shuitu
ST-11 Qishe
ST-12 Quepen

LI-20 Yingxiang
LI-19 Kouheliao
LI-18 Futu
LI-17 Tianding

SI-19 Tinggong
SI-18 Quanliao
SI-17 Tianrong
SI-16 Tianchuang

TB-23 Sizhukong
TB-22 Erheliao
TB-21 Ermen
TB-20 Jiaosun

TB-19 Luxi
TB-18 Chimai
TB-17 Yifeng
TB-16 Tianyou

EX-HN-14 Yiming
GB-1 Tongziliao
GB-2 Tinghui
GB-3 Shangguan
GB-4 Hanyan
GB-5 Xuanlu
GB-6 Xuanli
GB-7 Qubin
GB-8 Shuaigu
GB-9 Tianchong
GB-10 Fubai
GB-11 Touqiaoyin
GB-12 Wangu
GB-13 Benshen
GB-14 Yangbai
GB-15 Toulinqi
GB-16 Muchuang
GB-17 Zhengying
GB-18 Chengling
GB-19 Naokong
GB-20 Fengchi

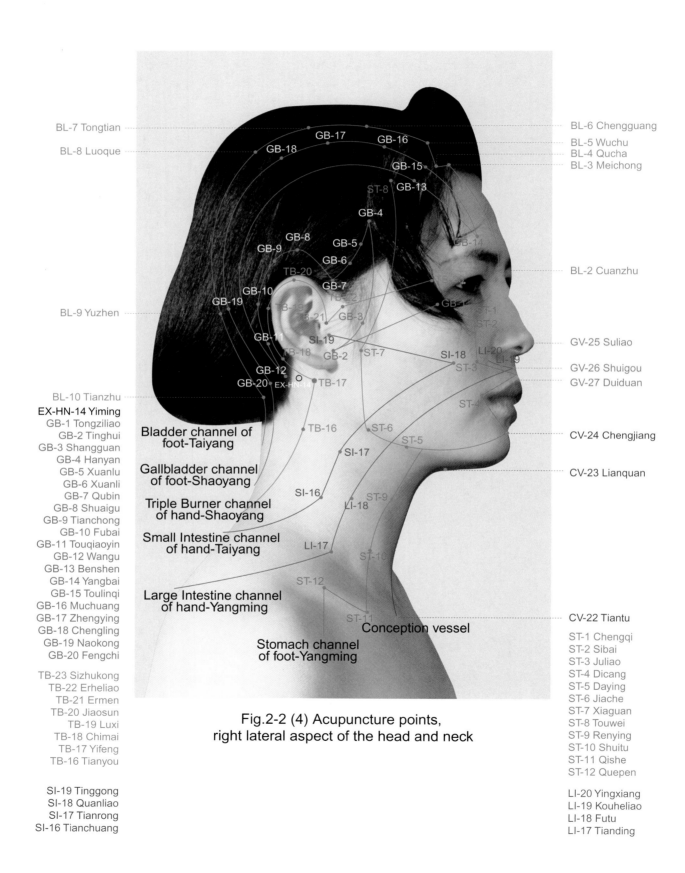

BL-7 Tongtian
BL-8 Luoque

BL-9 Yuzhen

BL-10 Tianzhu
EX-HN-14 Yiming
GB-1 Tongziliao
GB-2 Tinghui
GB-3 Shangguan
GB-4 Hanyan
GB-5 Xuanlu
GB-6 Xuanli
GB-7 Qubin
GB-8 Shuaigu
GB-9 Tianchong
GB-10 Fubai
GB-11 Touqiaoyin
GB-12 Wangu
GB-13 Benshen
GB-14 Yangbai
GB-15 Toulinqi
GB-16 Muchuang
GB-17 Zhengying
GB-18 Chengling
GB-19 Naokong
GB-20 Fengchi

TB-23 Sizhukong
TB-22 Erheliao
TB-21 Ermen
TB-20 Jiaosun
TB-19 Luxi
TB-18 Chimai
TB-17 Yifeng
TB-16 Tianyou

SI-19 Tinggong
SI-18 Quanliao
SI-17 Tianrong
SI-16 Tianchuang

BL-6 Chengguang
BL-5 Wuchu
BL-4 Qucha
BL-3 Meichong

BL-2 Cuanzhu

GV-25 Suliao
GV-26 Shuigou
GV-27 Duiduan

CV-24 Chengjiang

CV-23 Lianquan

CV-22 Tiantu
ST-1 Chengqi
ST-2 Sibai
ST-3 Juliao
ST-4 Dicang
ST-5 Daying
ST-6 Jiache
ST-7 Xiaguan
ST-8 Touwei
ST-9 Renying
ST-10 Shuitu
ST-11 Qishe
ST-12 Quepen

LI-20 Yingxiang
LI-19 Kouheliao
LI-18 Futu
LI-17 Tianding

Bladder channel of foot-Taiyang

Gallbladder channel of foot-Shaoyang

Triple Burner channel of hand-Shaoyang

Small Intestine channel of hand-Taiyang

Large Intestine channel of hand-Yangming

Conception vessel

Stomach channel of foot-Yangming

Fig.2-2 (4) Acupuncture points,
right lateral aspect of the head and neck

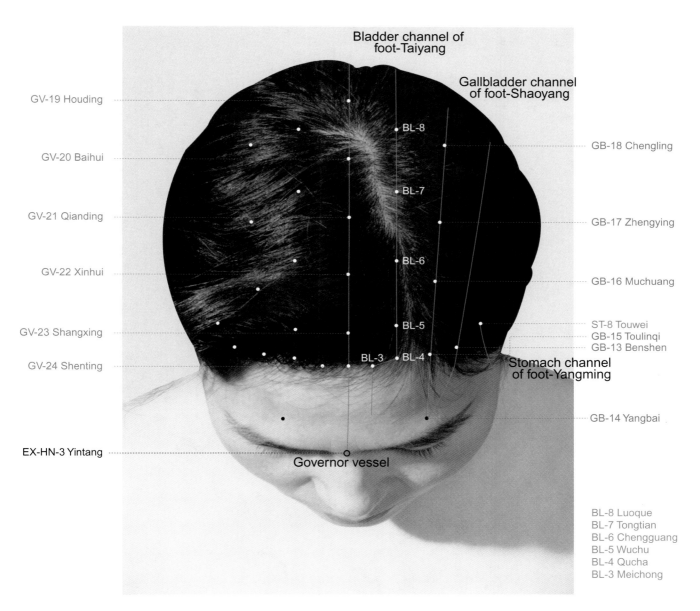

Bladder channel of foot-Taiyang

Gallbladder channel of foot-Shaoyang

GV-19 Houding

GV-20 Baihui

GV-21 Qianding

GV-22 Xinhui

GV-23 Shangxing

GV-24 Shenting

EX-HN-3 Yintang

BL-8

BL-7

BL-6

BL-5

BL-3 · BL-4

Governor vessel

GB-18 Chengling

GB-17 Zhengying

GB-16 Muchuang

ST-8 Touwei
GB-15 Toulinqi
GB-13 Benshen

Stomach channel of foot-Yangming

GB-14 Yangbai

BL-8 Luoque
BL-7 Tongtian
BL-6 Chengguang
BL-5 Wuchu
BL-4 Qucha
BL-3 Meichong

Fig.2-2 (5) Acupuncture points on the vertex

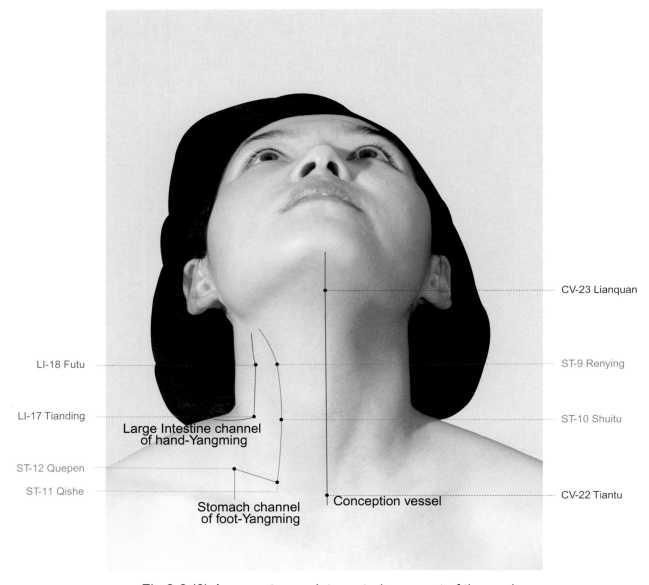

LI-18 Futu

LI-17 Tianding

Large Intestine channel
of hand-Yangming

ST-12 Quepen

ST-11 Qishe

Stomach channel
of foot-Yangming

Conception vessel

CV-23 Lianquan

ST-9 Renying

ST-10 Shuitu

CV-22 Tiantu

Fig.2-2 (6) Acupuncture points, anterior aspect of the neck

FIGURES OF ACUPUNCTURE POINTS ON THE ARM AND HAND

LU-10 Yuji
LU-9 Taiyuan
LU-8 Jingqu
LU-7 Lieque
LU-6 Kongzui
LU-5 Chize
LU-4 Xiabai
LU-3 Tianfu

PC-9 Zhongchong
PC-8 Laogong
PC-7 Daling
PC-6 Neiguan
PC-5 Jianshi
PC-4 Ximen
PC-3 Quze
PC-2 Tianquan

HT-8 Shaofu
HT-7 Shenmen
HT-6 Yinxi
HT-5 Tongli
HT-4 Lingdao
HT-3 Shaohai
HT-2 Qingling
HT-1 Jiquan

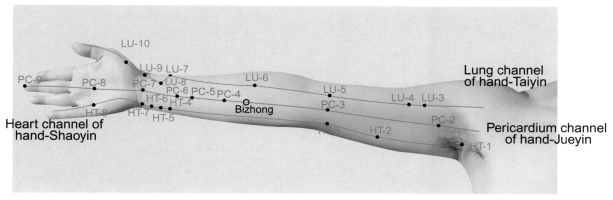

Fig.2-3 (1) Acupuncture points, anterior aspect of the arm and hand

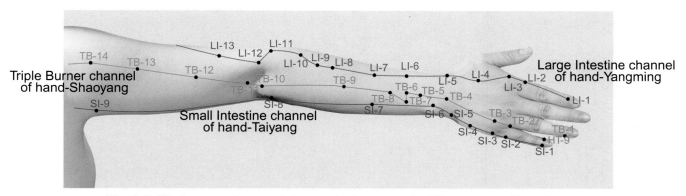

Fig.2-3 (2) Acupuncture points, posterior aspect of the arm and hand

LI-13 Shouwuli
LI-12 Zhouliao
LI-11 Quchi
LI-10 Shousanli
LI-9 Shanglian
LI-8 Xialian
LI-7 Wenliu
LI-6 Pianli
LI-5 Yangxi
LI-4 Hegu
LI-3 Sanjian
LI-2 Erjian
LI-1 Shangyang

TB-14 Jianliao
TB-13 Naohui
TB-12 Xiaoluo
TB-11 Qinglengyuan
TB-10 Tianjing
TB-9 Sidu
TB-8 Sanyangluo
TB-7 Huizong
TB-6 Zhigou
TB-5 Waiguan
TB-4 Yangchi
TB-3 Zhongzhu
TB-2 Yemen
TB-1 Guanchong

SI-9 Jianzhen
SI-8 Xiaohai
SI-7 Zhizheng
SI-6 Yanglao
SI-5 Yanggu
SI-4 Wangu
SI-3 Houxi
SI-2 Qiangu
SI-1 Shaoze

HT-9 Shaochong

LI-1 Shangyang
LI-2 Erjian
LI-3 Sanjian
LI-4 Hegu

LU-11 Shaoshang
LU-6 Kongzui
LU-5 Chize
LU-4 Xiabai
LU-3 Tianfu

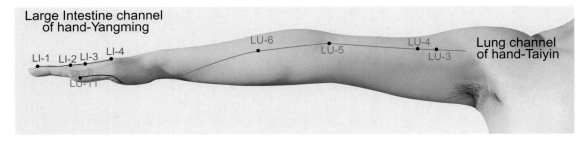

Fig.2-3 (3) Acupuncture points, radial aspect of the arm and hand

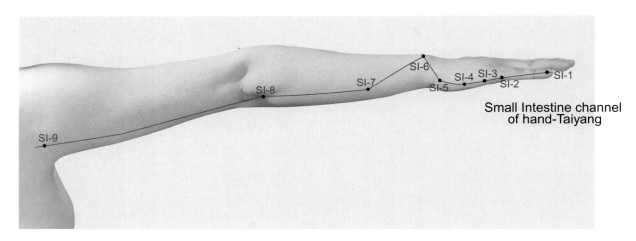

Fig.2-3 (4) Acupuncture points, ulnar aspect of the arm and hand

SI-9 Jianzhen
SI-8 Xiaohai
SI-7 Zhizheng
SI-6 Yanglao
SI-5 Yanggu
SI-4 Wangu
SI-3 Houxi
SI-2 Qiangu
SI-1 Shaoze

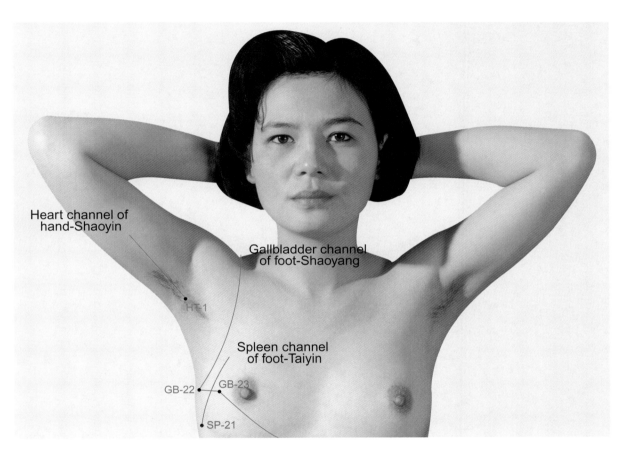

Fig.2-3 (5) Acupuncture points in the axillary region

HT-1 Jiquan   GB-22 Yuanye   SP-21 Dabao

GB-23 Zhejin

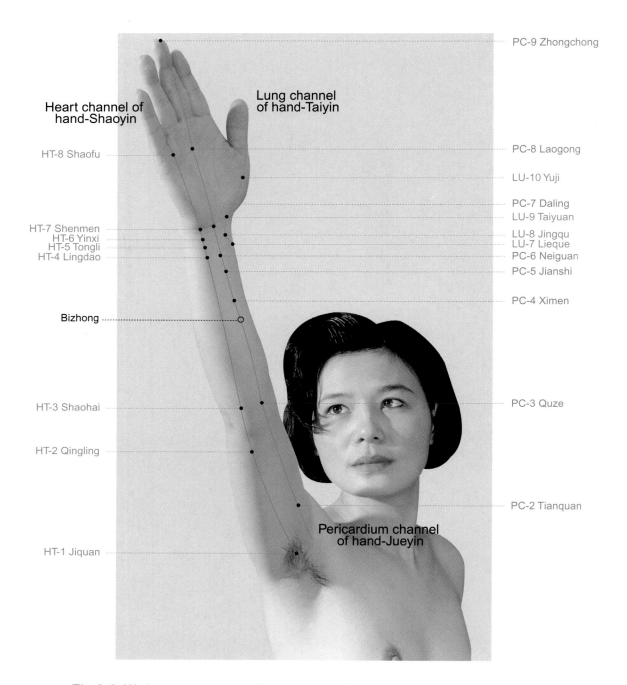

Fig.2-3 (6) Acupuncture points, anteromedial aspect of the arm and hand

LU-5 Chize
LU-4 Xiabai
LU-3 Tianfu

PC-3 Quze
PC-2 Tianquan

HT-3 Shaohai
HT-2 Qingling
HT-1 Jiquan

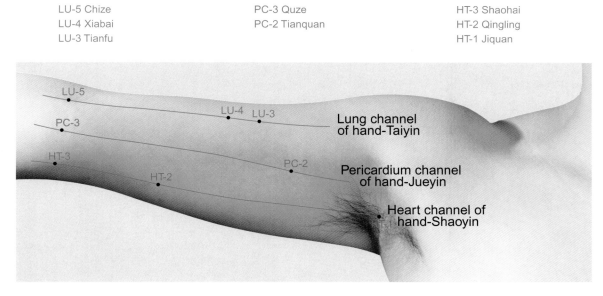

Fig.2-3 (7) Acupuncture points, anterior aspect of the upper arm

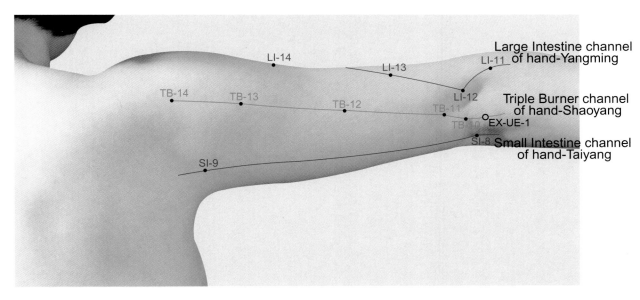

Fig.2-3 (8) Acupuncture points, posterior aspect of the upper arm

LI-14 Binao
LI-13 Shouwuli
LI-12 Zhouliao
LI-11 Quchi

TB-14 Jianliao
TB-13 Naohui
TB-12 Xiaoluo
TB-11 Qinglengyuan
TB-10 Tianjing

SI-9 Jianzhen
SI-8 Xiaohai

EX-UE-1 Zhoujian

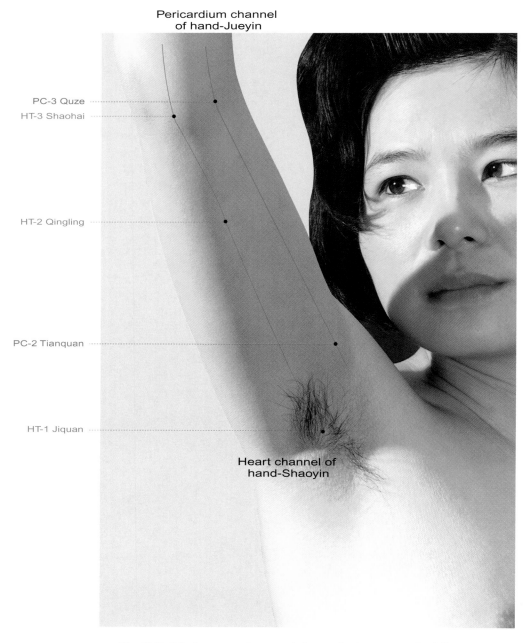

Fig.2-3 (9) Acupuncture points, anterior aspect of the upper arm

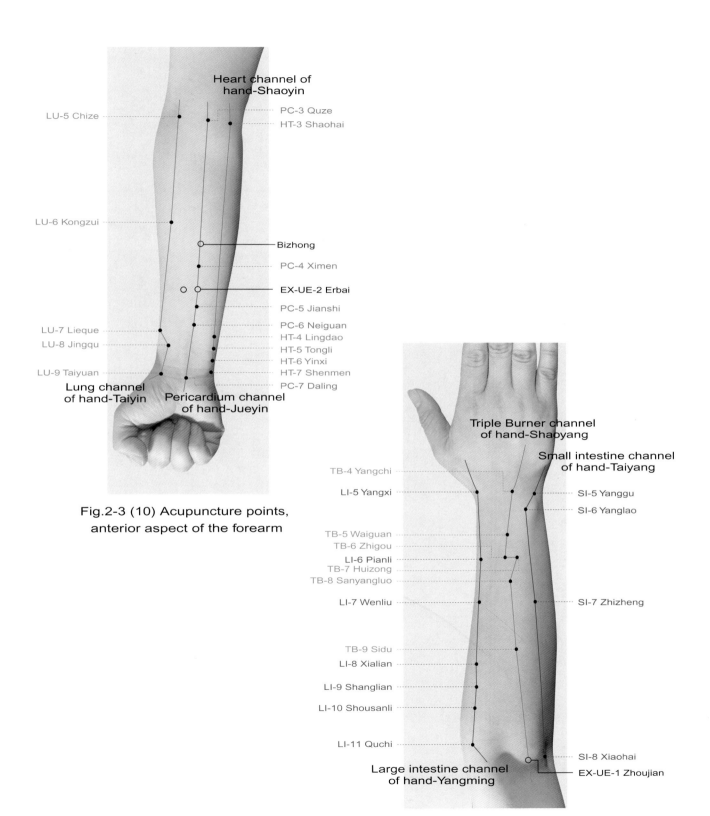

Heart channel of hand-Shaoyin

LU-5 Chize
PC-3 Quze
HT-3 Shaohai

LU-6 Kongzui

Bizhong
PC-4 Ximen
EX-UE-2 Erbai
PC-5 Jianshi
PC-6 Neiguan
LU-7 Lieque
HT-4 Lingdao
LU-8 Jingqu
HT-5 Tongli
HT-6 Yinxi
LU-9 Taiyuan
HT-7 Shenmen
PC-7 Daling

Lung channel of hand-Taiyin
Pericardium channel of hand-Jueyin

Fig.2-3 (10) Acupuncture points, anterior aspect of the forearm

Triple Burner channel of hand-Shaoyang

Small intestine channel of hand-Taiyang

TB-4 Yangchi
LI-5 Yangxi
SI-5 Yanggu
SI-6 Yanglao

TB-5 Waiguan
TB-6 Zhigou
LI-6 Pianli
TB-7 Huizong
TB-8 Sanyangluo

LI-7 Wenliu
SI-7 Zhizheng

TB-9 Sidu
LI-8 Xialian

LI-9 Shanglian

LI-10 Shousanli

LI-11 Quchi
SI-8 Xiaohai
EX-UE-1 Zhoujian

Large intestine channel of hand-Yangming

Fig.2-3 (11) Acupuncture points, posterior aspect of the forearm

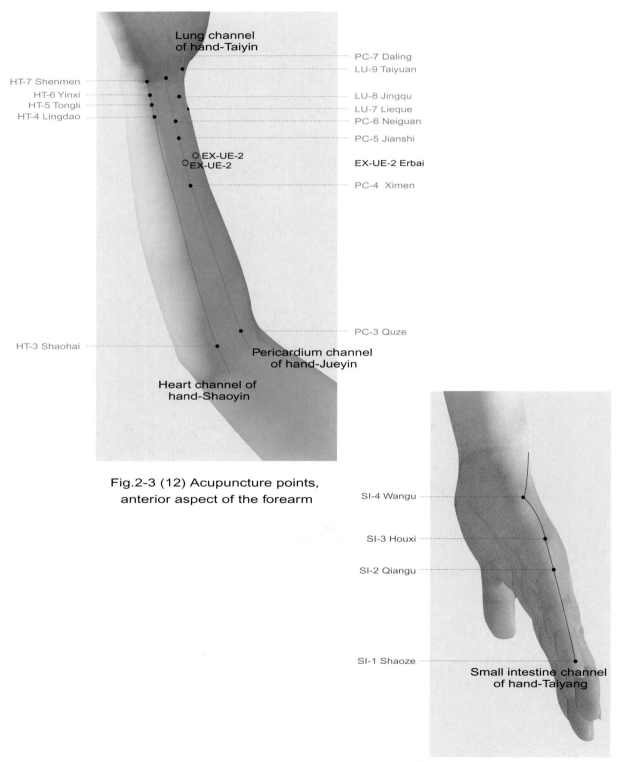

Lung channel
of hand-Taiyin

PC-7 Daling
LU-9 Taiyuan

HT-7 Shenmen

LU-8 Jingqu

HT-6 Yinxi
HT-5 Tongli
HT-4 Lingdao

LU-7 Lieque
PC-6 Neiguan

PC-5 Jianshi

EX-UE-2
EX-UE-2

EX-UE-2 Erbai

PC-4 Ximen

PC-3 Quze

HT-3 Shaohai

Pericardium channel
of hand-Jueyin

Heart channel of
hand-Shaoyin

Fig.2-3 (12) Acupuncture points,
anterior aspect of the forearm

SI-4 Wangu

SI-3 Houxi

SI-2 Qiangu

SI-1 Shaoze

Small intestine channel
of hand-Taiyang

Fig.2-3 (13) Acupuncture points,
posteromedial aspect of the hand

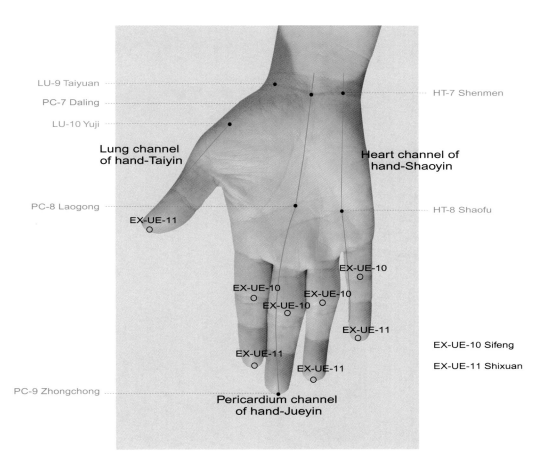

Fig.2-3 (14) Acupuncture points on the palm

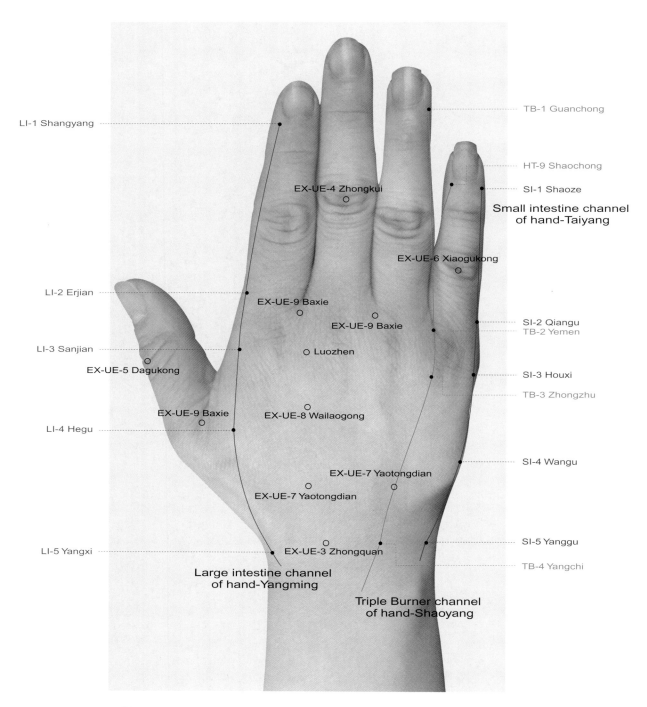

Fig.2-3 (15) Acupuncture points on the dorsum of the hand

FIGURES OF ACUPUNCTURE POINTS ON THE LEG AND FOOT

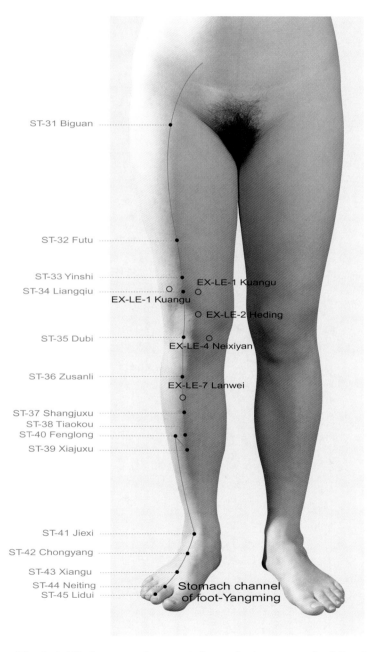

ST-31 Biguan

ST-32 Futu

ST-33 Yinshi

ST-34 Liangqiu

EX-LE-1 Kuangu

EX-LE-1 Kuangu

EX-LE-2 Heding

ST-35 Dubi

EX-LE-4 Neixiyan

ST-36 Zusanli

EX-LE-7 Lanwei

ST-37 Shangjuxu
ST-38 Tiaokou
ST-40 Fenglong
ST-39 Xiajuxu

ST-41 Jiexi

ST-42 Chongyang

ST-43 Xiangu
ST-44 Neiting
ST-45 Lidui

Stomach channel
of foot-Yangming

Fig.2-4 (1) Acupuncture points, anterior aspect of the leg and foot

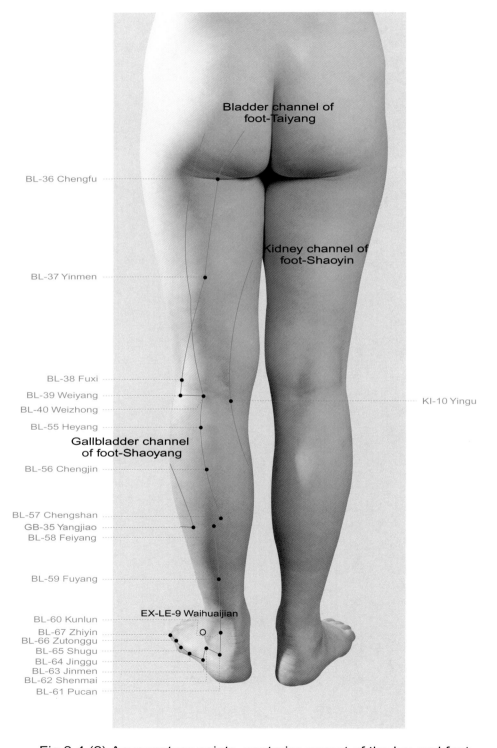

Fig.2-4 (2) Acupuncture points, posterior aspect of the leg and foot

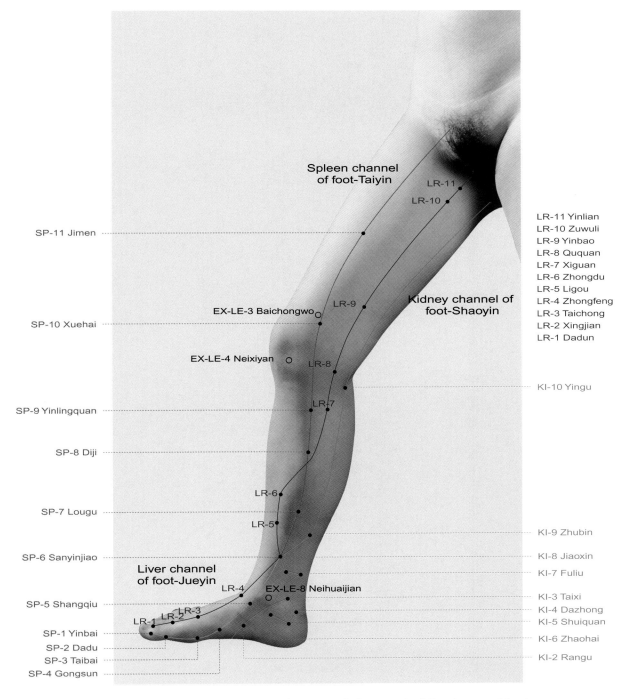

Spleen channel
of foot-Taiyin

LR-11
LR-10

SP-11 Jimen

Kidney channel of
foot-Shaoyin

EX-LE-3 Baichongwo   LR-9

SP-10 Xuehai

EX-LE-4 Neixiyan   LR-8

SP-9 Yinlingquan

LR-7

SP-8 Diji

LR-6

SP-7 Lougu

LR-5

SP-6 Sanyinjiao

Liver channel
of foot-Jueyin

LR-4   EX-LE-8 Neihuaijian

SP-5 Shangqiu

LR-3
LR-2
LR-1

SP-1 Yinbai
SP-2 Dadu
SP-3 Taibai
SP-4 Gongsun

LR-11 Yinlian
LR-10 Zuwuli
LR-9 Yinbao
LR-8 Ququan
LR-7 Xiguan
LR-6 Zhongdu
LR-5 Ligou
LR-4 Zhongfeng
LR-3 Taichong
LR-2 Xingjian
LR-1 Dadun

KI-10 Yingu

KI-9 Zhubin

KI-8 Jiaoxin

KI-7 Fuliu

KI-3 Taixi
KI-4 Dazhong
KI-5 Shuiquan

KI-6 Zhaohai

KI-2 Rangu

Fig.2-4 (3) Acupuncture points, medial aspect of the leg and foot

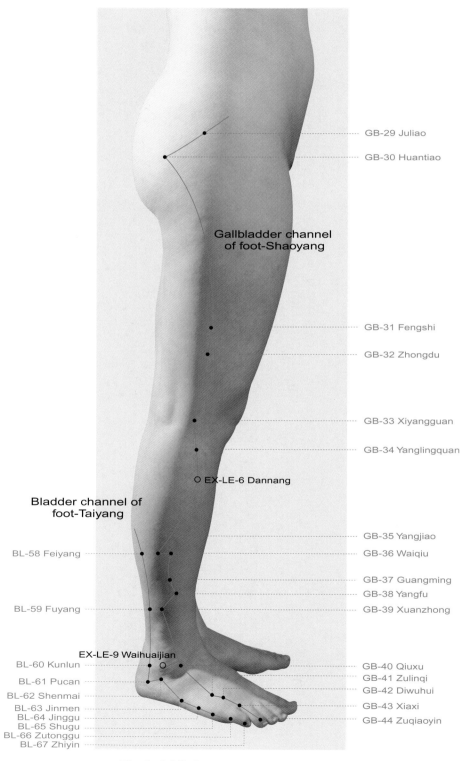

Gallbladder channel
of foot-Shaoyang

GB-29 Juliao

GB-30 Huantiao

GB-31 Fengshi

GB-32 Zhongdu

GB-33 Xiyangguan

GB-34 Yanglingquan

EX-LE-6 Dannang

Bladder channel of
foot-Taiyang

GB-35 Yangjiao

BL-58 Feiyang

GB-36 Waiqiu

GB-37 Guangming

GB-38 Yangfu

BL-59 Fuyang

GB-39 Xuanzhong

EX-LE-9 Waihuaijian

BL-60 Kunlun

GB-40 Qiuxu

BL-61 Pucan

GB-41 Zulinqi

BL-62 Shenmai

GB-42 Diwuhui

BL-63 Jinmen

GB-43 Xiaxi

BL-64 Jinggu

GB-44 Zuqiaoyin

BL-65 Shugu

BL-66 Zutonggu

BL-67 Zhiyin

Fig.2-4 (4) Acupuncture points,
lateral aspect of the leg and foot

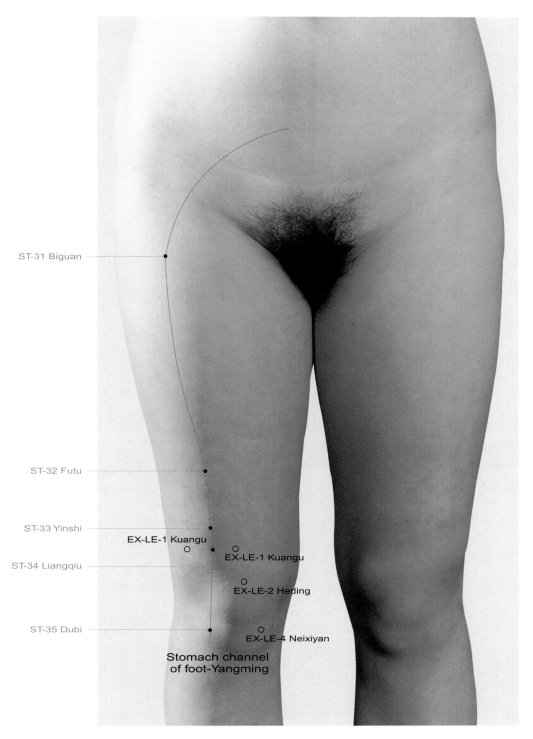

Fig.2-4 (5) Acupuncture points, anterior aspect of the thigh

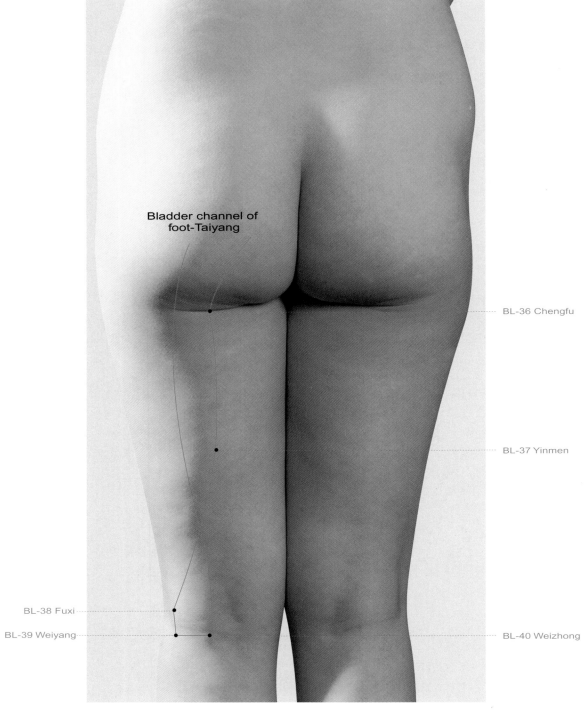

Fig.2-4 (6) Acupuncture points, posterior aspect of the thigh

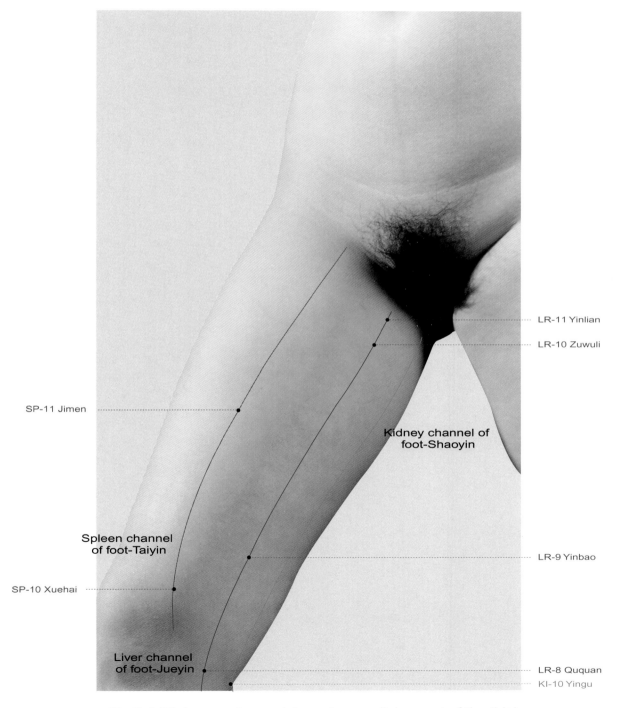

Fig.2-4 (7) Acupuncture points, anteromedial aspect of the thigh

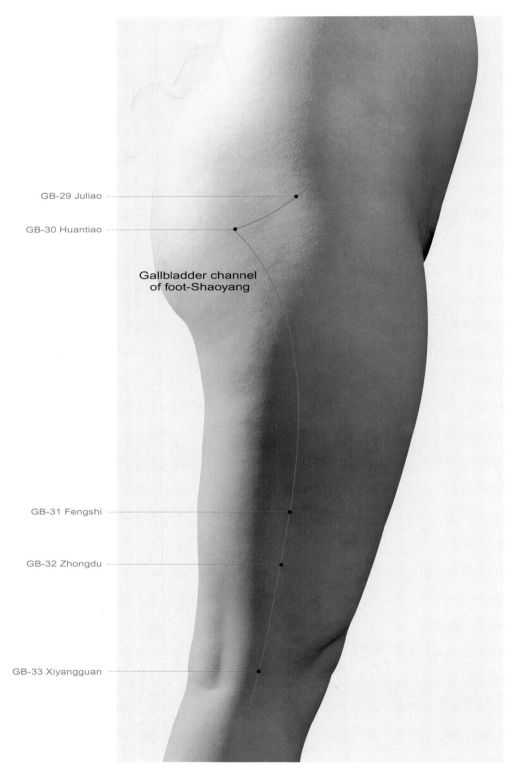

GB-29 Juliao

GB-30 Huantiao

Gallbladder channel of foot-Shaoyang

GB-31 Fengshi

GB-32 Zhongdu

GB-33 Xiyangguan

Fig.2-4 (8) Acupuncture points, lateral aspect of the thigh

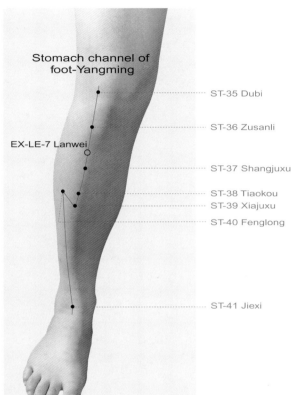

Stomach channel of
foot-Yangming

ST-35 Dubi

ST-36 Zusanli

EX-LE-7 Lanwei

ST-37 Shangjuxu

ST-38 Tiaokou
ST-39 Xiajuxu
ST-40 Fenglong

ST-41 Jiexi

Fig.2-4 (9) Acupuncture points,
anterior aspect of the lower leg

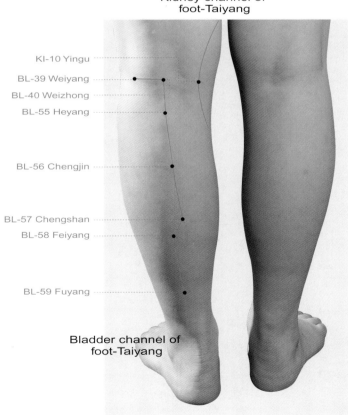

Kidney channel of
foot-Taiyang

KI-10 Yingu

BL-39 Weiyang

BL-40 Weizhong

BL-55 Heyang

BL-56 Chengjin

BL-57 Chengshan

BL-58 Feiyang

BL-59 Fuyang

Bladder channel of
foot-Taiyang

Fig.2-4 (10) Acupuncture points,
posterior aspect of the lower leg

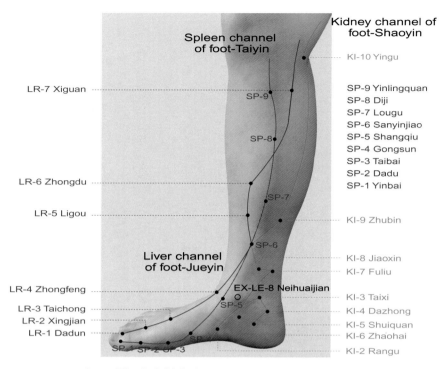

Spleen channel
of foot-Taiyin

Kidney channel of
foot-Shaoyin

KI-10 Yingu

LR-7 Xiguan

SP-9

SP-9 Yinlingquan
SP-8 Diji
SP-7 Lougu
SP-6 Sanyinjiao
SP-5 Shangqiu
SP-4 Gongsun
SP-3 Taibai
SP-2 Dadu
SP-1 Yinbai

SP-8

LR-6 Zhongdu

SP-7

LR-5 Ligou

KI-9 Zhubin

SP-6

Liver channel
of foot-Jueyin

KI-8 Jiaoxin
KI-7 Fuliu

LR-4 Zhongfeng

EX-LE-8 Neihuaijian

SP-5

KI-3 Taixi

LR-3 Taichong
LR-2 Xingjian
LR-1 Dadun

KI-4 Dazhong
KI-5 Shuiquan
KI-6 Zhaohai
KI-2 Rangu

SP-4 SP-2 SP-3

Fig.2-4 (11) Acupuncture points,
medial aspect of the lower leg

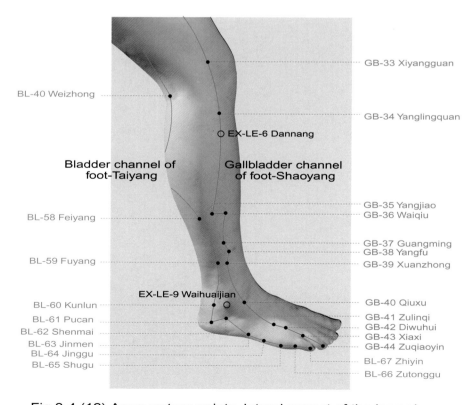

GB-33 Xiyangguan

BL-40 Weizhong

GB-34 Yanglingquan

EX-LE-6 Dannang

Bladder channel of
foot-Taiyang

Gallbladder channel
of foot-Shaoyang

GB-35 Yangjiao
GB-36 Waiqiu

BL-58 Feiyang

GB-37 Guangming
GB-38 Yangfu
GB-39 Xuanzhong

BL-59 Fuyang

EX-LE-9 Waihuaijian

GB-40 Qiuxu

BL-60 Kunlun
BL-61 Pucan
BL-62 Shenmai
BL-63 Jinmen
BL-64 Jinggu
BL-65 Shugu

GB-41 Zulinqi
GB-42 Diwuhui
GB-43 Xiaxi
GB-44 Zuqiaoyin

BL-67 Zhiyin
BL-66 Zutonggu

Fig.2-4 (12) Acupuncture points, lateral aspect of the lower leg

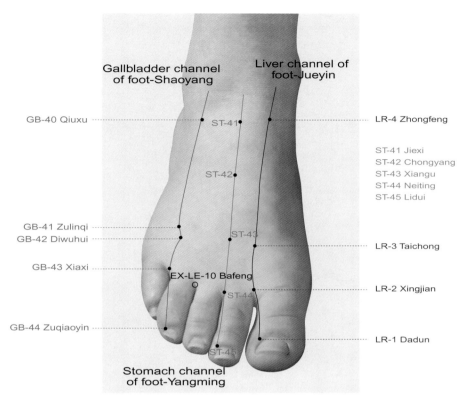

Gallbladder channel
of foot-Shaoyang

Liver channel of
foot-Jueyin

GB-40 Qiuxu

ST-41

LR-4 Zhongfeng

ST-41 Jiexi
ST-42 Chongyang
ST-43 Xiangu
ST-44 Neiting
ST-45 Lidui

ST-42

GB-41 Zulinqi
GB-42 Diwuhui

ST-43

LR-3 Taichong

GB-43 Xiaxi

EX-LE-10 Bafeng

ST-44

LR-2 Xingjian

GB-44 Zuqiaoyin

LR-1 Dadun

ST-45

Stomach channel
of foot-Yangming

Fig.2-4 (13) Acupuncture points
on the dorsum of the foot

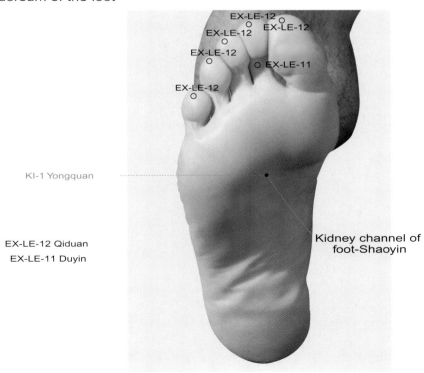

EX-LE-12
EX-LE-12
EX-LE-12
EX-LE-12
EX-LE-11
EX-LE-12

KI-1 Yongquan

EX-LE-12 Qiduan
EX-LE-11 Duyin

Kidney channel of
foot-Shaoyin

Fig.2-4 (14) Acupuncture points on the sole of the foot

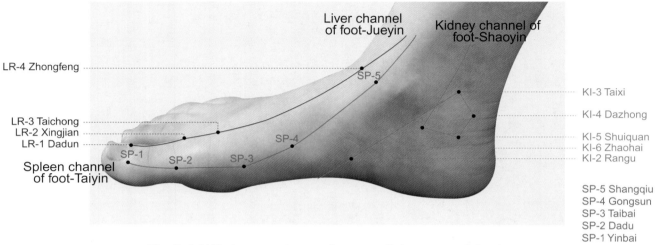

Liver channel of foot-Jueyin

Kidney channel of foot-Shaoyin

LR-4 Zhongfeng

SP-5

LR-3 Taichong
LR-2 Xingjian
LR-1 Dadun

SP-4

Spleen channel of foot-Taiyin

SP-1
SP-2
SP-3

KI-3 Taixi
KI-4 Dazhong
KI-5 Shuiquan
KI-6 Zhaohai
KI-2 Rangu

SP-5 Shangqiu
SP-4 Gongsun
SP-3 Taibai
SP-2 Dadu
SP-1 Yinbai

Fig.2-4 (15) Acupuncture points, medial aspect of the foot

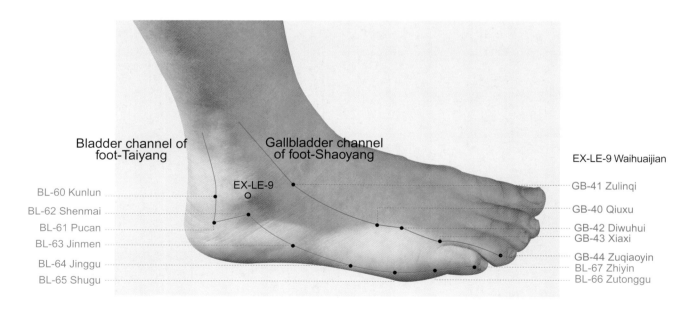

Bladder channel of foot-Taiyang

Gallbladder channel of foot-Shaoyang

EX-LE-9 Waihuaijian

BL-60 Kunlun

EX-LE-9

BL-62 Shenmai

BL-61 Pucan

BL-63 Jinmen

BL-64 Jinggu

BL-65 Shugu

GB-41 Zulinqi

GB-40 Qiuxu

GB-42 Diwuhui
GB-43 Xiaxi

GB-44 Zuqiaoyin
BL-67 Zhiyin
BL-66 Zutonggu

Fig.2-4 (16) Acupuncture points, lateral aspect of the foot

EAR ACUPUNCTURE POINTS

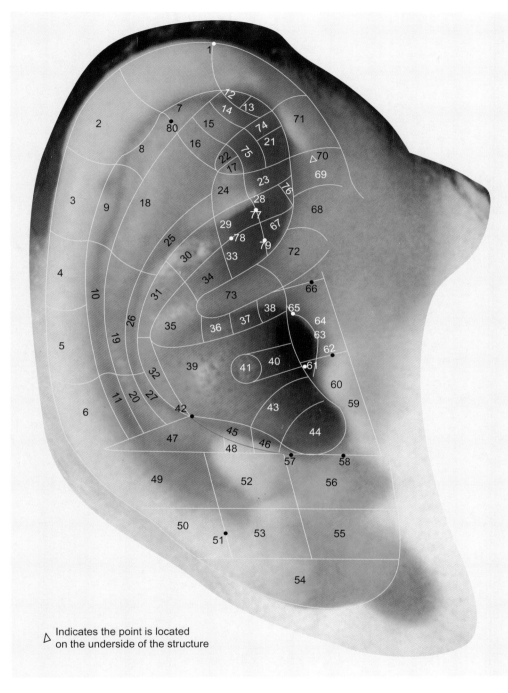

19. Thoracic vertebrae
20. Cervical vertebrae
21. Uterus
22. Ear Shenmen
23. Sciatic nerve
24. Buttock
25. Abdomen
26. Chest
27. Neck
28. Bladder
29. Kidney
30. Pancreas and gallbladder
31. Liver
32. Spleen
33. Small intestine
34. Duodenum
35. Stomach
36. Cardia
37. Esophagus
38. Mouth
39. Lung
40. Trachea
41. Heart
42. Brain stem
43. Triple Burner
44. Endocrine
45. Subcortex
46. Forehead
47. Occiput
48. Temple
49. Jaw
50. Internal ear
51. Cheek
52. Tongue
53. Eye
54. Tonsil
55. Anterior to lobe
56. Tooth
57. Posterior to intertragus
58. Anterior to intertragus
59. Medial to tragus
60. Internal nose
61. Adrenal gland
62. External nose
63. Superior to tragus
64. Throat (on underside of point)
65. Apex of tragus
66. External ear
67. Large intestine
68. Urethra
69. External genitalia
70. Sympathetic region
71. Hemorrhoids
72. Rectum
73. Middle ear
74. Superior triangular fossa
75. Middle triangular fossa
76. Angle of superior concha
77. Ureter
78. Middle superior concha
79. Appendix
80. Allergy

△ Indicates the point is located on the underside of the structure

1. Ear apex	7. Finger	13. Heel
2. Darwin's tubercle	8. Wrist	14. Ankle
3. Helix$_1$	9. Elbow	15. Knee
4. Helix$_2$	10. Shoulder	16. Hip
5. Helix$_3$	11. Clavicle	17. Pelvic cavity
6. Helix$_4$	12. Toe	18. Lumbosacral vertebrae

Fig.2-5 (1) Acupuncture points on the anterior lateral side of the auricle

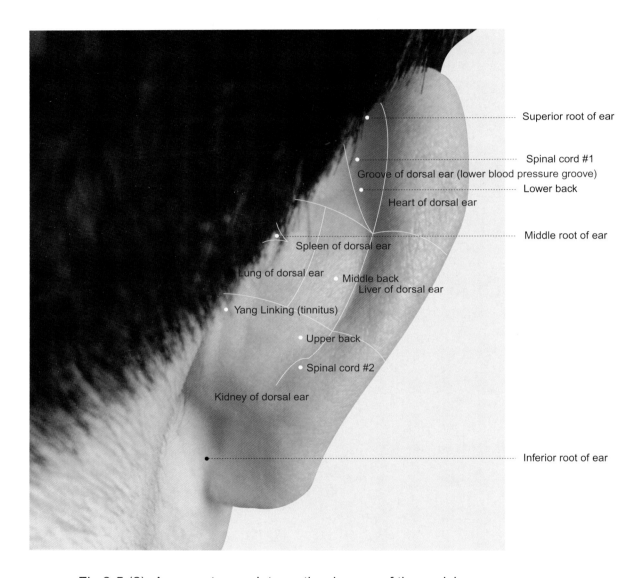

Superior root of ear

Spinal cord #1

Groove of dorsal ear (lower blood pressure groove)

Lower back

Heart of dorsal ear

Middle root of ear

Spleen of dorsal ear

Lung of dorsal ear   Middle back

Liver of dorsal ear

Yang Linking (tinnitus)

Upper back

Spinal cord #2

Kidney of dorsal ear

Inferior root of ear

Fig.2-5 (2) Acupuncture points on the dorsum of the auricle

3 Acupuncture points (sagittal section, left side)

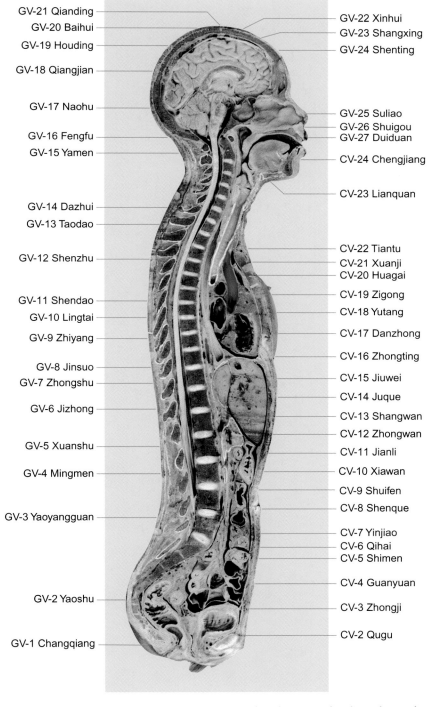

GV-21 Qianding
GV-20 Baihui
GV-19 Houding
GV-18 Qiangjian
GV-17 Naohu
GV-16 Fengfu
GV-15 Yamen
GV-14 Dazhui
GV-13 Taodao
GV-12 Shenzhu
GV-11 Shendao
GV-10 Lingtai
GV-9 Zhiyang
GV-8 Jinsuo
GV-7 Zhongshu
GV-6 Jizhong
GV-5 Xuanshu
GV-4 Mingmen
GV-3 Yaoyangguan
GV-2 Yaoshu
GV-1 Changqiang

GV-22 Xinhui
GV-23 Shangxing
GV-24 Shenting
GV-25 Suliao
GV-26 Shuigou
GV-27 Duiduan
CV-24 Chengjiang
CV-23 Lianquan
CV-22 Tiantu
CV-21 Xuanji
CV-20 Huagai
CV-19 Zigong
CV-18 Yutang
CV-17 Danzhong
CV-16 Zhongting
CV-15 Jiuwei
CV-14 Juque
CV-13 Shangwan
CV-12 Zhongwan
CV-11 Jianli
CV-10 Xiawan
CV-9 Shuifen
CV-8 Shenque
CV-7 Yinjiao
CV-6 Qihai
CV-5 Shimen
CV-4 Guanyuan
CV-3 Zhongji
CV-2 Qugu

Fig.3-1 (1) Conception and Governor vessel points on the head, neck and trunk

GV-21 Qianding

GV-20 Baihui

GV-19 Houding

GV-18 Qiangjian

GV-17 Naohu

GV-16 Fengfu

GV-15 Yamen

GV-14 Dazhui

GV-13 Taodao

GV-12 Shenzhu

GV-11 Shendao

GV-10 Lingtai

GV-9 Zhiyang

GV-22 Xinhui

GV-23 Shangxing

GV-24 Shenting

GV-25 Suliao

GV-26 Shuigou

GV-27 Duiduan

CV-24 Chengjiang

CV-23 Lianquan

CV-22 Tiantu

CV-21 Xuanji

CV-20 Huagai

CV-19 Zigong

CV-18 Yutang

CV-17 Danzhong

CV-16 Zhongting

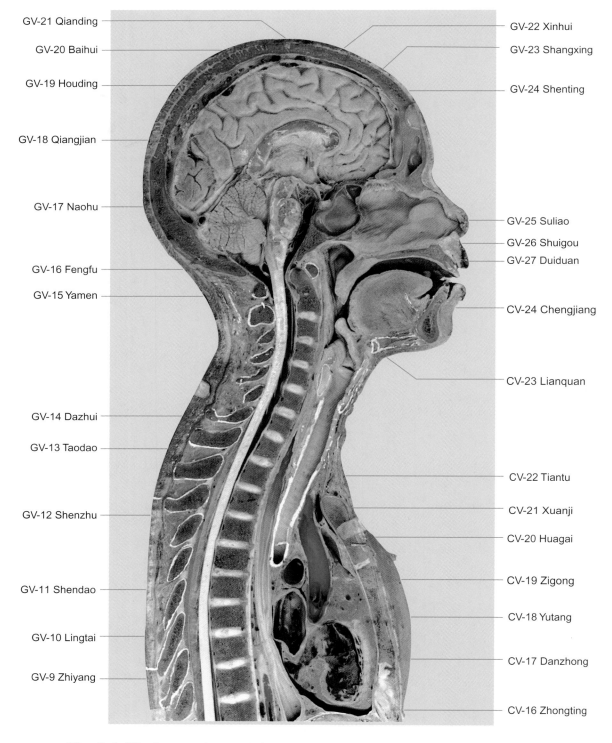

Fig. 3-1 (2) Conception and Governor vessel points on the upper trunk

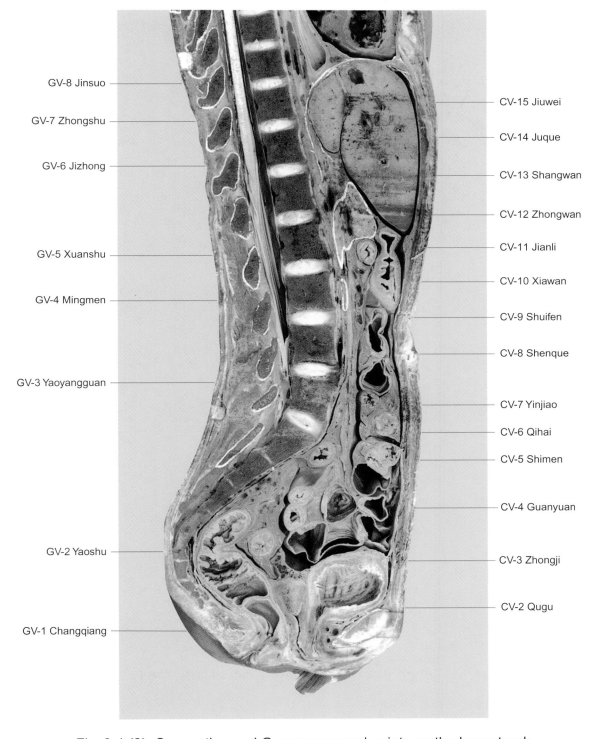

GV-8 Jinsuo

GV-7 Zhongshu

GV-6 Jizhong

GV-5 Xuanshu

GV-4 Mingmen

GV-3 Yaoyangguan

GV-2 Yaoshu

GV-1 Changqiang

CV-15 Jiuwei

CV-14 Juque

CV-13 Shangwan

CV-12 Zhongwan

CV-11 Jianli

CV-10 Xiawan

CV-9 Shuifen

CV-8 Shenque

CV-7 Yinjiao

CV-6 Qihai

CV-5 Shimen

CV-4 Guanyuan

CV-3 Zhongji

CV-2 Qugu

Fig. 3-1 (3)　Conception and Governor vessel points on the lower trunk

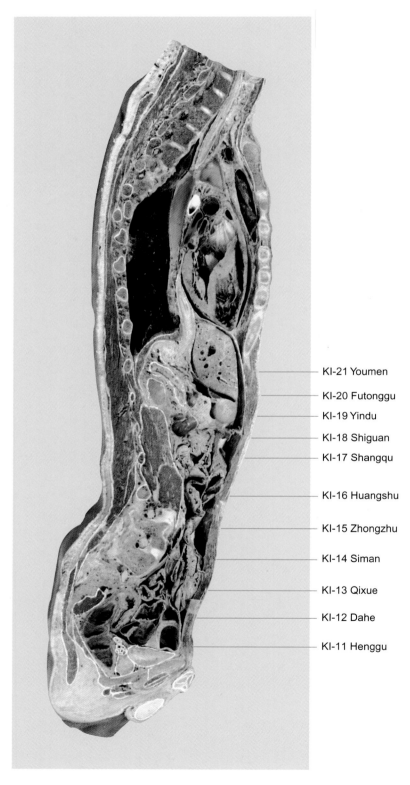

KI-21 Youmen
KI-20 Futonggu
KI-19 Yindu
KI-18 Shiguan
KI-17 Shangqu
KI-16 Huangshu
KI-15 Zhongzhu
KI-14 Siman
KI-13 Qixue
KI-12 Dahe
KI-11 Henggu

Fig. 3-2 (1) Abdominal points on the Kidney channel,
0.5 cun lateral to the anterior midline

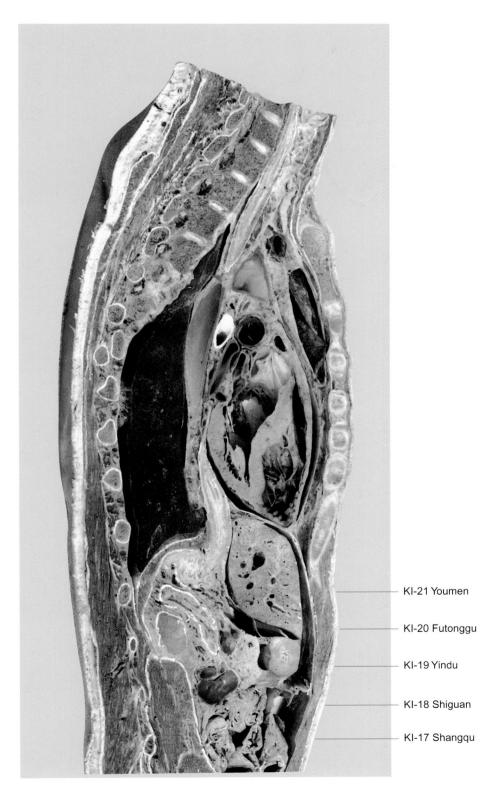

KI-21 Youmen

KI-20 Futonggu

KI-19 Yindu

KI-18 Shiguan

KI-17 Shangqu

Fig. 3-2 (2) Kidney channel points on the upper trunk,
0.5 cun lateral to the anterior midline

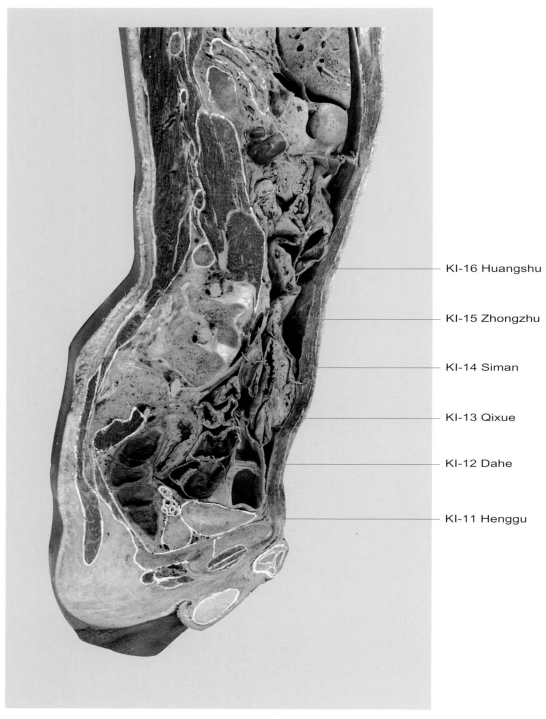

KI-16 Huangshu

KI-15 Zhongzhu

KI-14 Siman

KI-13 Qixue

KI-12 Dahe

KI-11 Henggu

Fig. 3-2 (3) Kidney channel points on the lower trunk,
0.5 cun lateral to the anterior midline

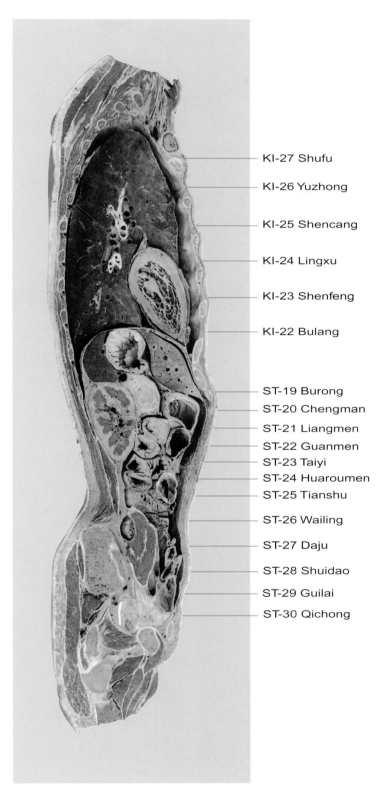

KI-27 Shufu

KI-26 Yuzhong

KI-25 Shencang

KI-24 Lingxu

KI-23 Shenfeng

KI-22 Bulang

ST-19 Burong
ST-20 Chengman
ST-21 Liangmen
ST-22 Guanmen
ST-23 Taiyi
ST-24 Huaroumen
ST-25 Tianshu

ST-26 Wailing

ST-27 Daju

ST-28 Shuidao

ST-29 Guilai

ST-30 Qichong

Fig. 3-3 (1) Points on the Kidney and Stomach channels,
2 cun lateral to the anterior midline

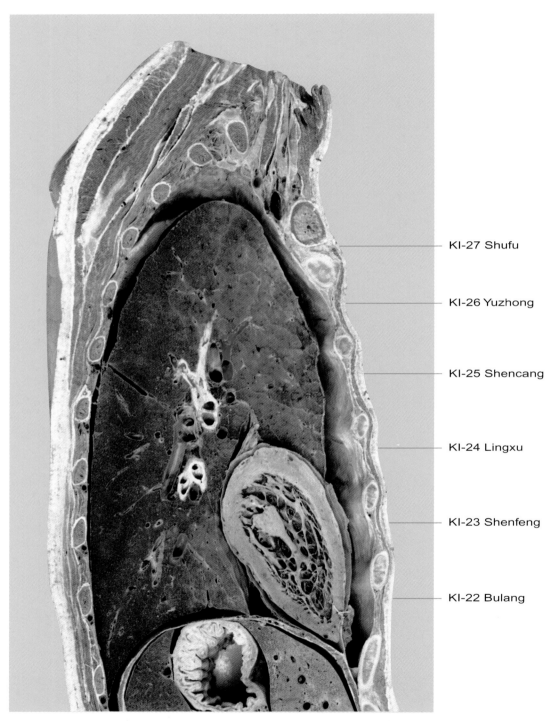

KI-27 Shufu

KI-26 Yuzhong

KI-25 Shencang

KI-24 Lingxu

KI-23 Shenfeng

KI-22 Bulang

Fig. 3-3 (2) Kidney channel points on the chest,
2 cun lateral to the anterior midline

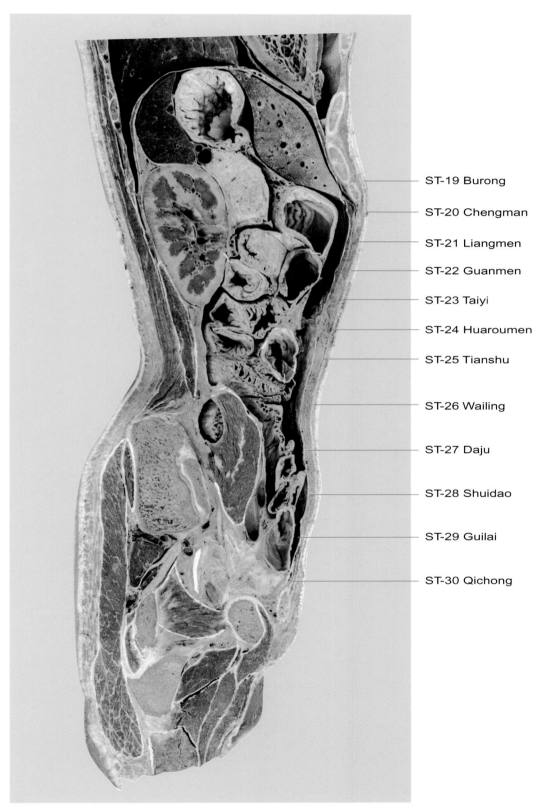

ST-19 Burong

ST-20 Chengman

ST-21 Liangmen

ST-22 Guanmen

ST-23 Taiyi

ST-24 Huaroumen

ST-25 Tianshu

ST-26 Wailing

ST-27 Daju

ST-28 Shuidao

ST-29 Guilai

ST-30 Qichong

Fig. 3-3 (3) Stomach channel points on the abdomen,
2 cun lateral to the anterior midline

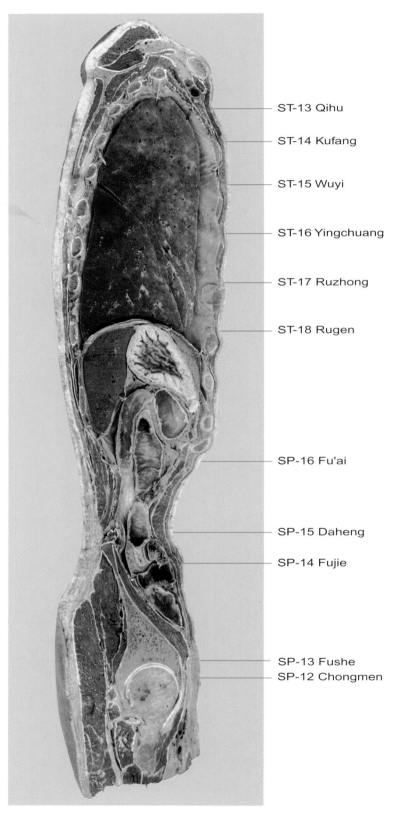

Fig. 3-4 (1) Points on the Stomach and Spleen channels,
4 cun lateral to the anterior midline
(except SP-12 Chongmen 3.5 cun lateral)

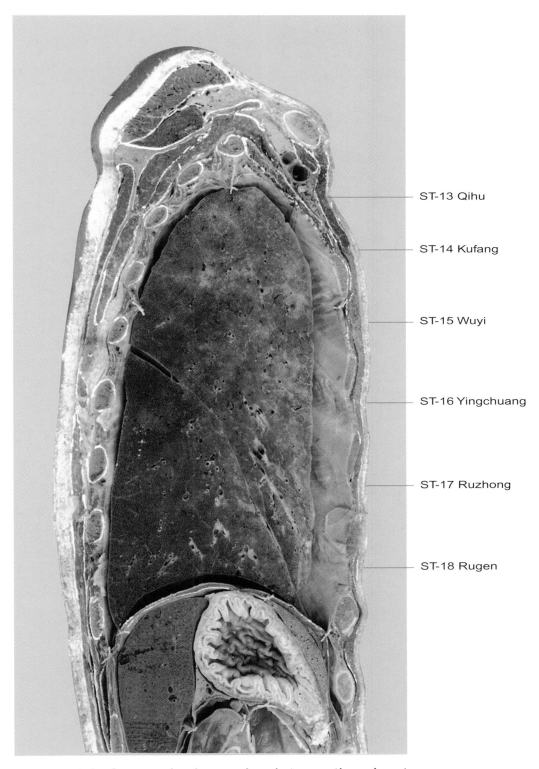

ST-13 Qihu

ST-14 Kufang

ST-15 Wuyi

ST-16 Yingchuang

ST-17 Ruzhong

ST-18 Rugen

Fig. 3-4 (2) Stomach channel points on the chest,
4 cun lateral to the anterior midline

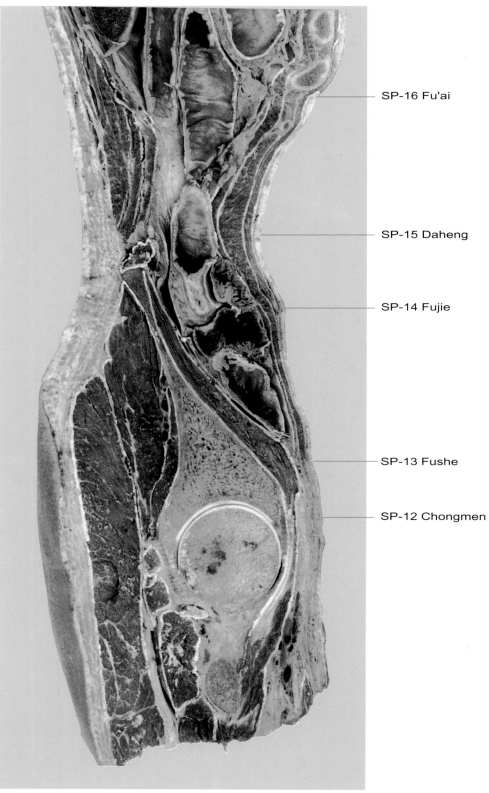

SP-16 Fu'ai

SP-15 Daheng

SP-14 Fujie

SP-13 Fushe

SP-12 Chongmen

Fig. 3-4 (3) Spleen channel points on the abdomen,
4 cun lateral to the anterior midline
(except SP-12 Chongmen, 3.5 cun lateral)

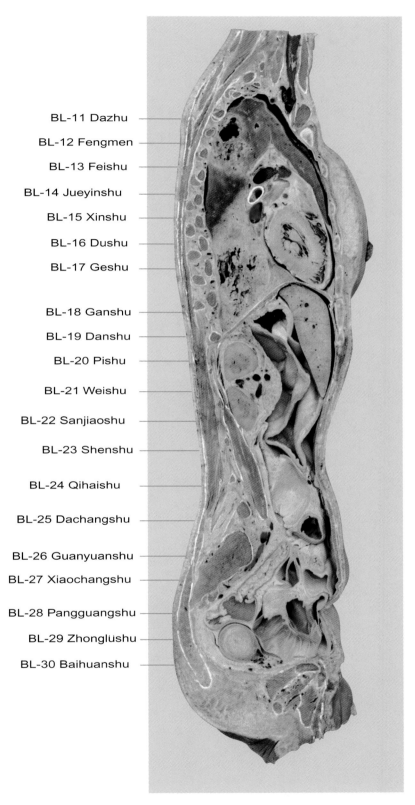

BL-11 Dazhu
BL-12 Fengmen
BL-13 Feishu
BL-14 Jueyinshu
BL-15 Xinshu
BL-16 Dushu
BL-17 Geshu

BL-18 Ganshu
BL-19 Danshu
BL-20 Pishu
BL-21 Weishu
BL-22 Sanjiaoshu
BL-23 Shenshu
BL-24 Qihaishu
BL-25 Dachangshu
BL-26 Guanyuanshu
BL-27 Xiaochangshu
BL-28 Pangguangshu
BL-29 Zhonglushu
BL-30 Baihuanshu

Fig. 3-5 (1) Points on the Bladder channel,
1.5 cun lateral to the posterior midline

BL-11 Dazhu

BL-12 Fengmen

BL-13 Feishu

BL-14 Jueyinshu

BL-15 Xinshu

BL-16 Dushu

BL-17 Geshu

BL-18 Ganshu

BL-19 Danshu

BL-20 Pishu

BL-21 Weishu

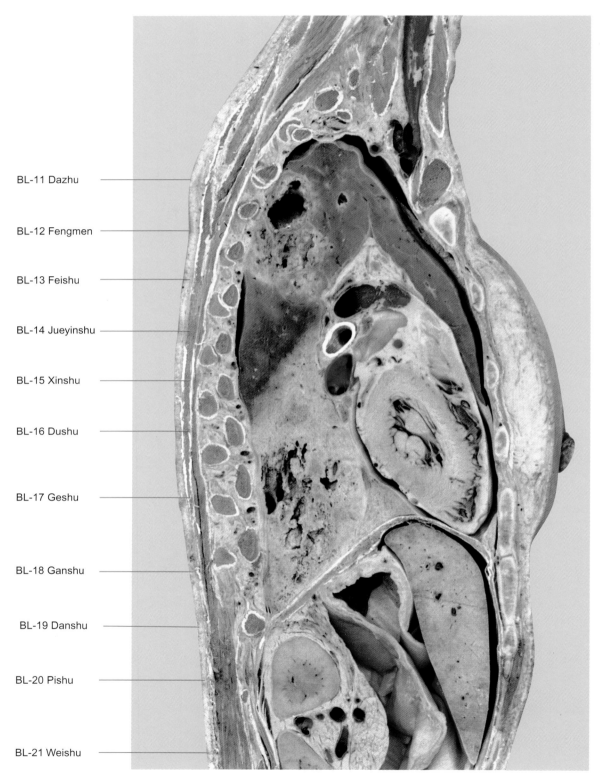

Fig. 3-5 (2) Bladder channel points on the upper back,
1. 5 cun lateral to the posterior midline

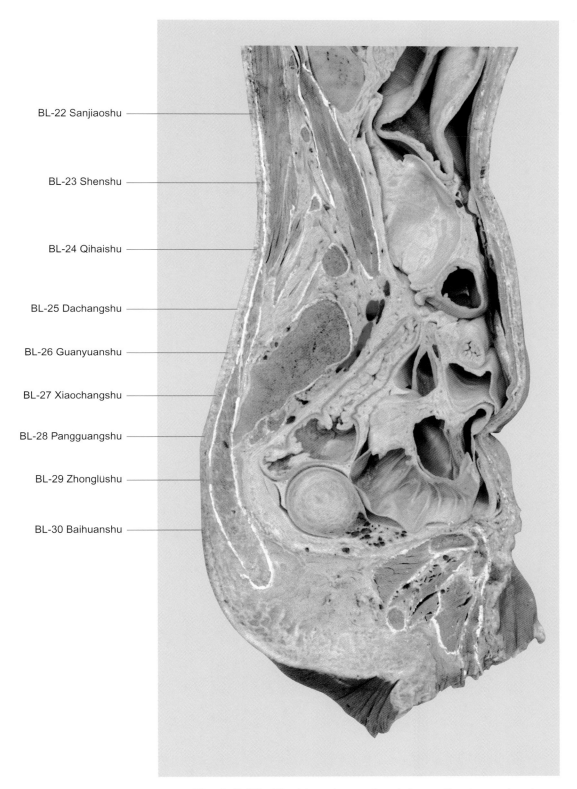

BL-22 Sanjiaoshu

BL-23 Shenshu

BL-24 Qihaishu

BL-25 Dachangshu

BL-26 Guanyuanshu

BL-27 Xiaochangshu

BL-28 Pangguangshu

BL-29 Zhonglüshu

BL-30 Baihuanshu

Fig. 3-5 (3) Bladder channel points on the lower back,
1.5 cun lateral to the posterior midline

BL-41 Fufen

BL-42 Pohu

BL-43 Gaohuang

BL-44 Shentang

BL-45 Yixi

BL-46 Geguan

BL-47 Hunmen

BL-48 Yanggang

BL-49 Yishe

BL-50 Weicang

BL-51 Huangmen

BL-52 Zhishi

BL-53 Baohuang

BL-54 Zhibian

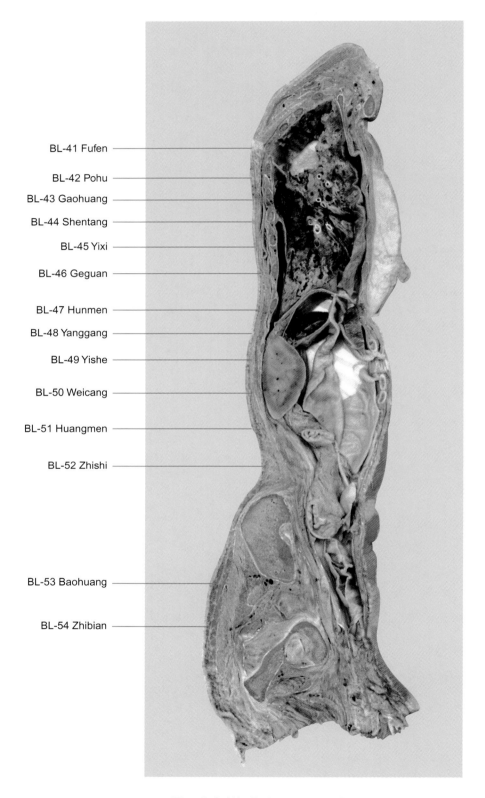

Fig. 3-6 (1) Points on the Bladder channel,
3 cun lateral to the posterior midline

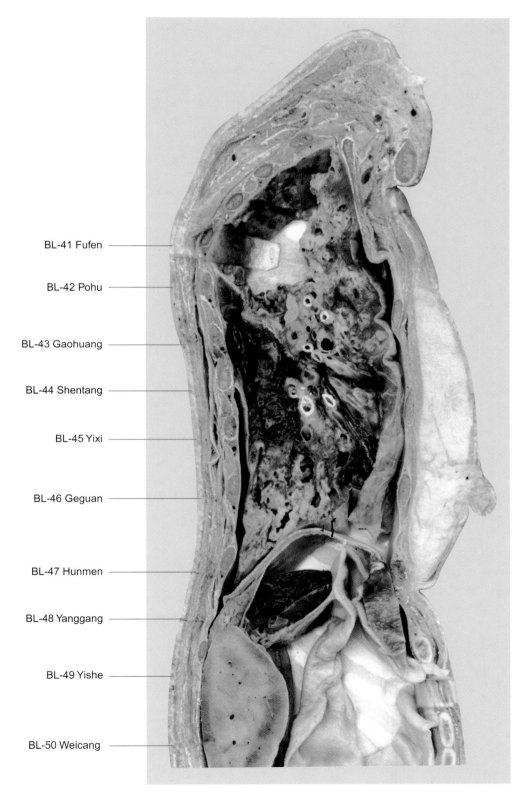

BL-41 Fufen

BL-42 Pohu

BL-43 Gaohuang

BL-44 Shentang

BL-45 Yixi

BL-46 Geguan

BL-47 Hunmen

BL-48 Yanggang

BL-49 Yishe

BL-50 Weicang

Fig. 3-6 (2) Bladder channel points on the upper back,
3 cun lateral to the posterior midline

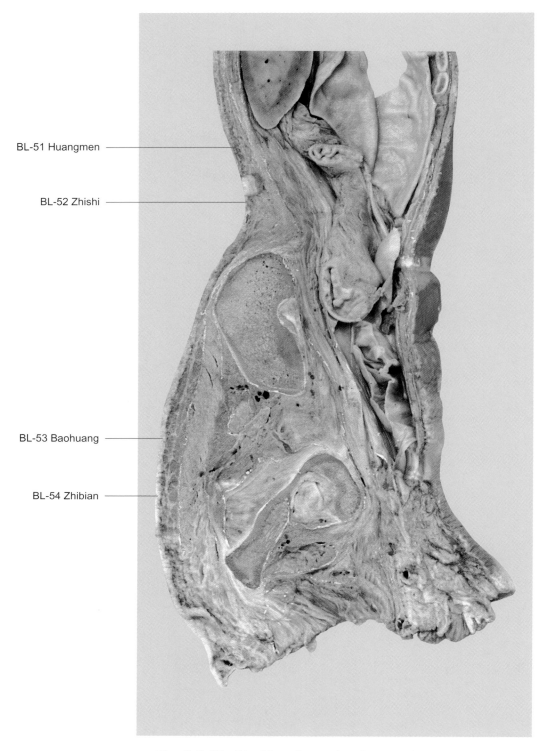

BL-51 Huangmen

BL-52 Zhishi

BL-53 Baohuang

BL-54 Zhibian

Fig. 3-6 (3) Bladder channel points on the lower back,
3 cun lateral to the posterior midline

4 Sectional figures of acupuncture points on the head, neck and trunk

ACUPUNCTURE POINTS ON THE HEAD AND NECK

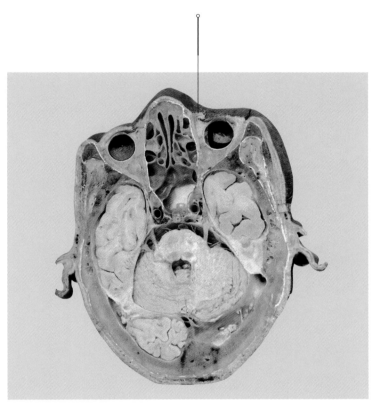

Fig. 4-1 (1) Transverse sectional figure of BL-1 Jingming

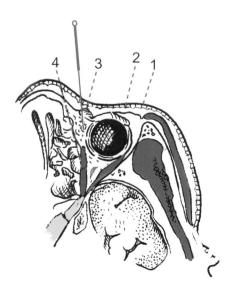

Transverse sectional figure of BL-1 Jingming (right)

BL-1 Jingming

Location 0.1 cun superior to the inner canthus of the eye.

Method Close the eye, push the eyeball to the lateral side and insert a filiform needle slowly and perpendicularly 0.3-0.5 cun along the orbital wall.

Actions Expels Wind, clears Heat and benefits the eyes.

Indications Conjunctivitis, myopia, hypermetropia, astigmatism, color blindness, optic neuritis, retinitis, glaucoma, mild cataract, corneal pigmentation, pterygium, and lacrimation.

Stratified anatomy 1. skin; 2. subcutaneous tissue; 3. orbicular muscle of eye; 4. point lies between the intermus muscle of the eye and the orbital lamina of the ethmoid bone.

Cautions The tip of needle at a depth of 19mm may injure the anterior ethmoidal artery and vein; at over 32mm, it may injure the paranasal choroidal or iridial artery; at 50mm, it may injure the optic nerve and ophthalmic artery along the optic foramen; at 51mm, it may injure the cavernous sinus or three layer meninges and cerebral temporal lobe.

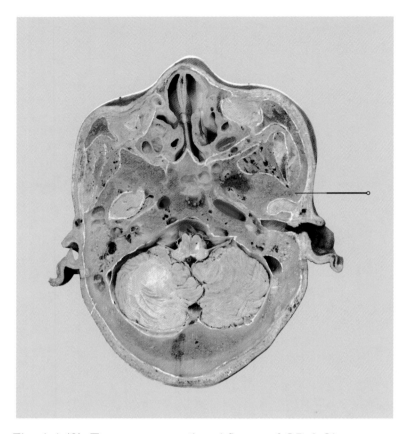

Fig. 4-1 (2) Transverse sectional figure of GB-3 Shangguan

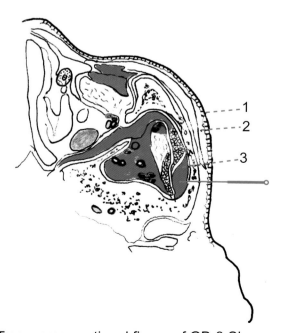

Transverse sectional figure of GB-3 Shangguan (right)

GB-3 Shangguan

Location Anterior to the ear, on the superior border of the zygomatic arch, directly superior to ST-7 Xiaguan.

Method Insert perpendicularly 0.5-0.8 cun.

Actions Expels Wind, invigorates the channels, alleviates pain, and benefits the ears.

Indications Tinnitus, deafness, otitis media, toothache, trismus, and facial paralysis.

Stratified anatomy 1. skin; 2. subcutaneous tissue; 3. temporal muscle.

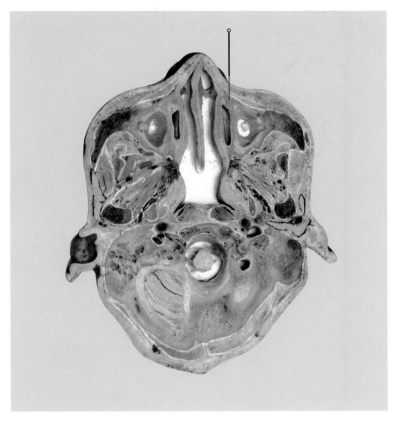

Fig. 4-1 (3) Transverse sectional figure of Bitong

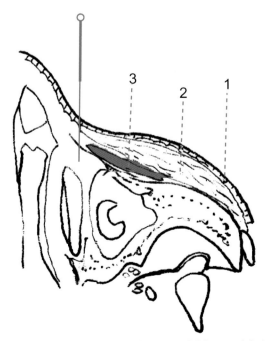

Transverse sectional figure of Bitong (right)

Bitong

Location At the highest point of the naso-labial groove.

Method Insert transversely 0.3-0.5 cun medio-superiorly.

Actions Benefits the nose.

Indications Rhinitis, nasal obstruction, pyogenic infection of the nose, allergic rhinitis, hypertrophic rhinitis, atrophic rhinitis, and nasal sinusitis.

Stratified anatomy 1. skin; 2. subcutaneous tissue; 3. levator muscle of upper lip and ala nasi.

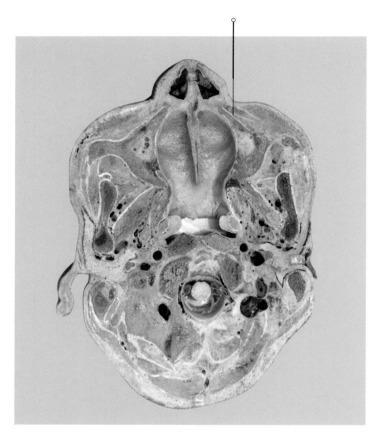

Fig. 4-1 (4) Transverse sectional figure of LI-20 Yingxiang

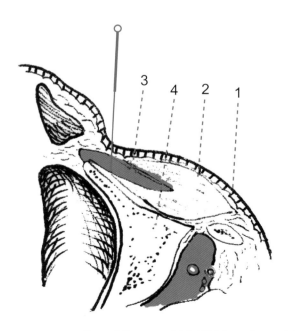

Transverse sectional figure of LI-20 Yingxiang (right)

LI-20 Yingxiang

Location In the upper border of the nasolabial groove, at the level of the midpoint of the lateral border of the ala nasi, 0.5 cun from the nostril.

Method Insert transversely toward Bitong 0.5-0.8 cun or toward ST-2 Sibai 0.5-1 cun, or insert perpendicularly 0.3-0.5 cun.

Actions Expels Wind and clears Heat, benefits the nose and opens the nasal passages.

Indications Rhinitis, nasal sinusitis, facial paralysis, and biliary ascariasis.

Stratified anatomy 1. skin; 2. subcutaneous tissue; 3. levator muscle of the upper lip; 4. maxillary bone.

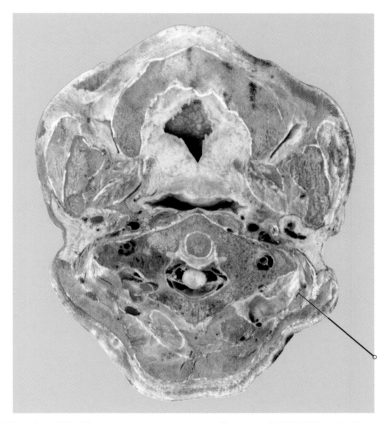

Fig. 4-1 (5) Transverse sectional figure of EX-HN-14 Yiming

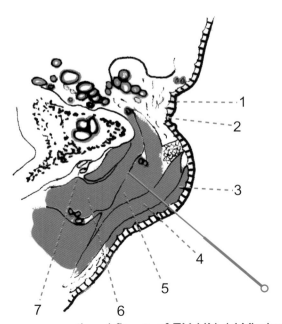

Transverse sectional figure of EX-HN-14 Yiming (right)

EX-HN-14 Yiming

Location 1 cun posterior to TB-17 Yifeng.

Method Insert perpendicularly 0.5-1 cun.

Actions Expels Wind, benefits the ears and eyes.

Indications Myopia, hypermetropia, early-stage cataract, schizophrenia, tinnitus, aphasia, headache, and vertigo.

Stratified anatomy 1. skin; 2. subcutaneous tissue; 3. sternocleidomastoid muscle; 4. splenius capitis muscle; 5. longissimus capitis muscle; 6. semispinalis capitis muscle; 7. vertebral artery.

Cautions Do not insert too deeply to avoid injuring the deep cervical artery and vein and the vertebral artery.

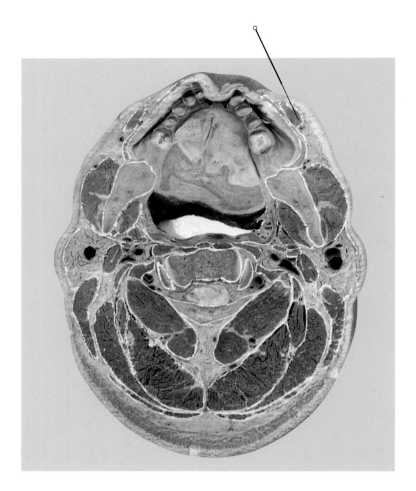

Fig. 4-1 (6) Transverse sectional figure of ST-4 Dicang

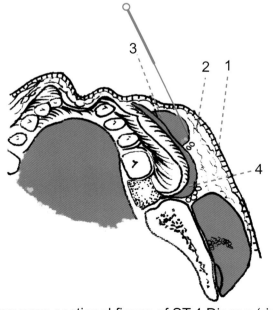

Transverse sectional figure of ST-4 Dicang (right)

ST-4 Dicang

Location 0.4 cun lateral to the corner of the mouth.

Method Insert obliquely 0.5-0.8 cun or transversely to join adjacent points.

Actions Expels Wind, invigorates the channels and alleviates pain.

Indications Facial paralysis and trigeminal neuralgia.

Stratified anatomy 1. skin; 2. subcutaneous tissue; 3. orbicular muscle of the mouth; 4. buccinator muscle.

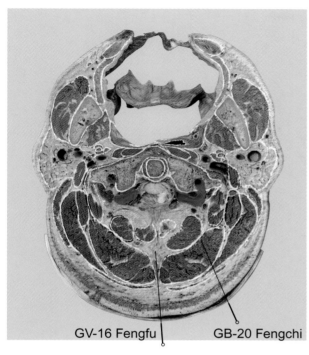

Fig. 4-1 (7) Transverse sectional figure of
GV-16 Fengfu and GB-20 Fengchi

GV-16 Fengfu

Location 1 cun directly superior to the midpoint of the posterior hairline in the depression just below the external occipital protuberance.

Method Insert perpendicularly or obliquely inferiorly 0.5-1 cun.

Actions Expels Wind, calms the Spirit, benefits the head and neck, and nourishes the Sea of Marrow.

Indications Stiffness and pain in the neck, numbness of the limbs, common cold, headache, apoplexy, and schizophrenia.

Stratified anatomy 1. skin; 2. subcutaneous tissue; 3. trapezius muscle; 6. semispinalis capitis muscle; 7. rectus capitis posterior major muscle; 9. nuchal ligament.

Cautions Do not insert the needle over 1.5 cun or it may injure the cerebellum, medullary bulb or posterior inferior cerebellar artery and cause serious damage.

GB-20 Fengchi

Location Directly inferior to the external occipital protuberance, in the depression lateral to GV-16 Fengfu, between the origins of the sternocleidomastoid and trapezius muscles.

Method Insert perpendicularly or obliquely toward the contralateral inner canthus 0.5-1 cun.

Actions Expels Wind, invigorates the channels, alleviates pain, and clears the sense organs.

Indications Common cold, vertigo, headache, stiffness and pain in the neck, ophthalmopathy, rhinitis, tinnitus, deafness, hypertension, epilepsy, hemiplegia, and encephalopathy.

Stratified anatomy 1. skin; 2. subcutaneous tissue; 3. trapezius muscle; 4. sternocleidomastoid muscle; 5. splenius capitis muscle; 6. semispinalis capitis muscle; 7. rectus capitis posterior major muscle medial to the needle; 8. capitis obliquus superior muscle lateral to the needle.

Cautions Do not insert the needle over 1.5 cun toward the contralateral outer canthus or it may injure the upper spinal cord or the lower part of the medullary bulb and cause serious damage.

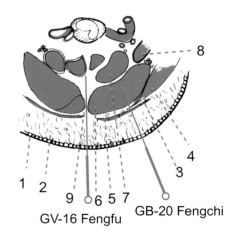

Transverse sectional figure of
GV-16 Fengfu and GB-20 Fengchi (right)

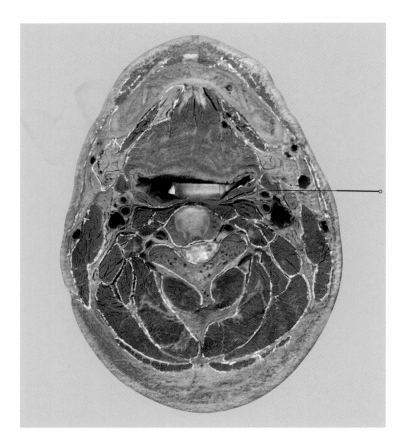

Fig. 4-1 (8) Transverse sectional figure of SI-17 Tianrong

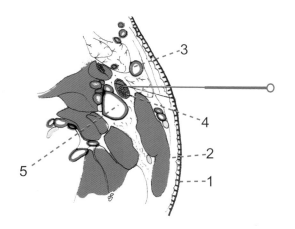

Transverse sectional figure
of SI-17 Tianrong (right)

SI-17 Tianrong

Location On the superior part of the lateral aspect of the neck, in the depression anterior to the sternocleidomastoid muscle and posterior to the mandible angle.

Method Insert perpendicularly 0.5-0.8 cun.

Actions Benefits the neck and throat, disperses swelling and bears counterflow Qi downward.

Indications Tonsillitis, laryngopharyngitis, stiffness, pain and swelling of the neck, and asthma.

Stratified anatomy 1. skin; 2. subcutaneous tissue; 3. facial artery; 4. digastric muscle tendon and stylohyoid muscle; 5. external carotid artery.

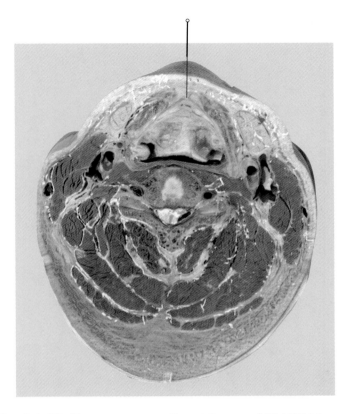

Fig. 4-1 (9) Transverse sectional figure of CV-23 Lianquan

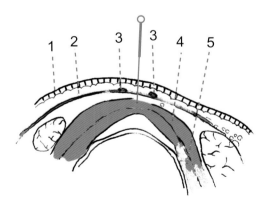

Transverse sectional figure of CV-23 Lianquan

CV-23 Lianquan

Location On the neck midline, superior to the thyrohyoid muscle, in the depression superior to the upper border of the hyoid bone.

Method Insert perpendicularly 0.3-0.5 cun.

Actions Bears Qi downward, stops coughing and benefits the tongue.

Indications Asthma, bronchitis, tonsillitis, aphonia, and paralysis of the muscles of the tongue.

Stratified anatomy 1. skin; 2. subcutaneous tissue; 3. point lies between the left and right anterior belly of the digastric muscle; 4. mylohyoid muscle; 5. geniohyoid muscle.

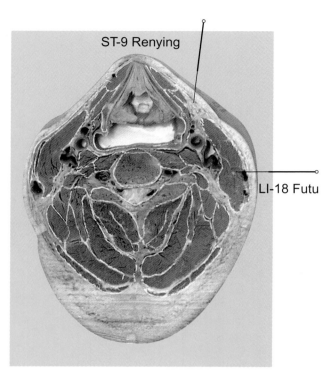

Fig. 4-1 (10) Transverse sectional figure of ST-9 Renying and LI-18 Futu

ST-9 Renying

Location In the carotid triangle, on the anterior border of the sternocleidomastoid muscle, 1.5 cun lateral to the laryngeal protuberance.

Method Avoiding the common carotid artery, insert perpendicularly 0.3-0.4 cun.

Actions Benefits the throat and neck, alleviates pain, regulates Qi and Blood.

Indications Hypertension, asthma, goiter, swelling and pain in the throat, and aphonia.

Stratified anatomy 1. skin; 2. subcutaneous tissue and platysma; 3. sternocleidomastoid muscle; 4. deep layer of cervical fascia; 5. constrictor muscle of the pharynx; 6. internal jugular vein, common carotid artery and branches, with adjacent vagus nerve.

Cautions Do not insert too deeply to avoid injuring the superior thyroid artery and vein and the common carotid artery.

LI-18 Futu

Location On the lateral side of the neck, 3 cun lateral to the laryngeal protuberance, between the sternal and clavicular heads of the sterno-cleidomastoid muscle.

Method Insert perpendicularly 0.5-1 cun.

Actions Benefits the throat and voice, stops coughing.

Indications Hoarseness, swelling and pain in the throat, cough, and dysphagia.

Stratified anatomy 1. skin; 2. subcutaneous tissue; 3. sternocleidomastoid muscle; 6. internal jugular vein, common carotid artery and branches, with adjacent vagus nerve.

Cautions Do not insert too deeply to avoid injuring the posterior border of the carotid sheath which contains the common carotid artery, the internal jugular vein, and the vagus nerve.

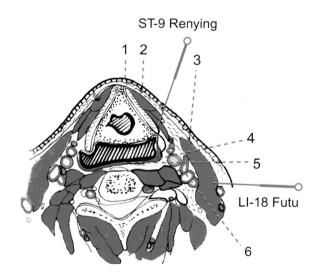

Transverse sectional figure of ST-9 Renying (right) and LI-18 Futu (right)

ST-1 Chengqi

Location With the eyes looking straight ahead, this point is directly below the pupil, between the eyeball and the infraorbital ridge.

Method Insert slowly and perpendicularly 0.3-0.5 cun along the infraorbital ridges.

Actions Expels Wind, clears Heat and benefits the eyes.

Indications Acute and chronic conjunctivitis, myopia, color blindness, glaucoma, optic neuritis, optic nerve atrophy, cataract, keratitis, and pigmentary degeneration of the retina.

Stratified anatomy 1. skin; 2. subcutaneous tissue; 3. orbicular muscle of the eye and levator muscle of the upper lip; 4. adipose body of the orbit; 5. inferior oblique muscle of the orbit.

Cautions Lifting and thrusting manipulation and deep insertion are contraindicated to avoid hematoma caused by injury to branches of the ophthalmic artery and veins.

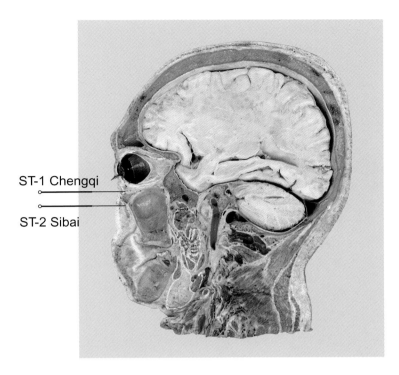

Fig. 4-1 (11) Sagittal sectional figure of ST-1 Chengqi and ST-2 Sibai

ST-2 Sibai

Location With the eyes looking straight ahead, this point is 1 cun directly below the pupil, in the depression of the infraorbital foramen.

Method Insert perpendicularly 0.2-0.3 cun.

Actions Expels Wind, clears Heat and benefits the eyes.

Indications Facial paralysis and spasm, trigeminal neuralgia, keratitis, myopia, nasal sinusitis, and biliary ascariasis.

Stratified anatomy 1. skin; 2. subcutaneous tissue; 3. orbicular muscle of the eye and levator muscle of the upper lip.

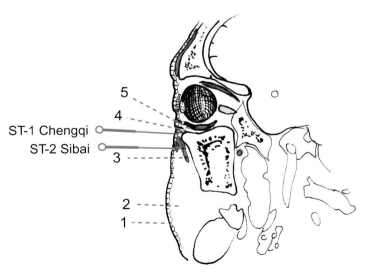

Sagittal sectional figure of ST-1 Chengqi (right) and ST-2 Sibai (right)

ACUPUNCTURE POINTS ON THE TRUNK

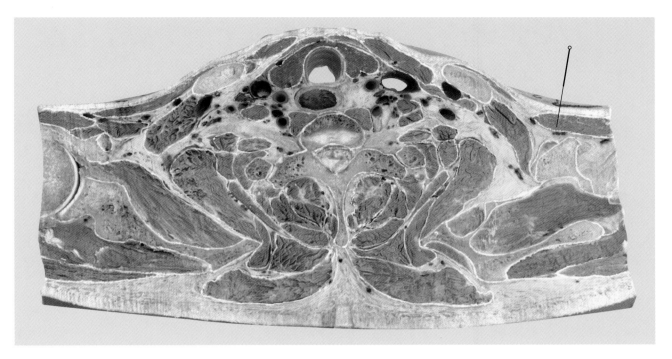

Fig. 4-2 (1) Transverse sectional figure of LU-2 Yunmen

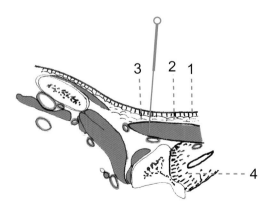

Transverse sectional figure
of LU-2 Yunmen (right)

LU-2 Yunmen

Location At the lateral inferior part of the clavicle 6 cun lateral to the anterior midline in the depression medial to the coracoid process of the scapula.

Method Insert obliquely 0.5 cun.

Actions Clears Heat, bears Lung Qi downward and disperses fullness from the chest.

Indications Cough, chest pain, chest distress, asthma, and scapulohumeral periarthritis (frozen shoulder).

Stratified anatomy 1. skin; 2. subcutaneous tissue; 3. deltoid muscle; 4. coracoclavicular ligament.

Cautions Do not insert deeply medially to avoid injuring the lung.

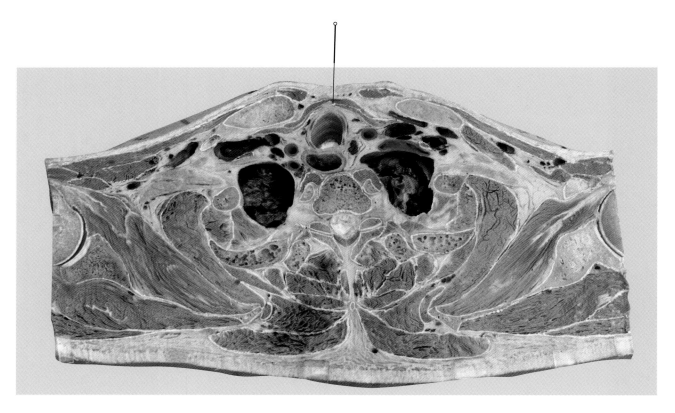

Fig. 4-2 (2) Transverse sectional figure of CV-22 Tiantu

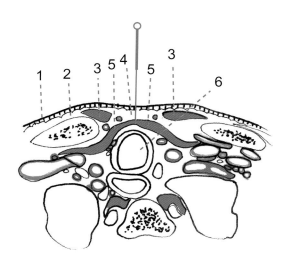

Transverse sectional figure
of CV-22 Tiantu

CV-22 Tiantu

Location On the anterior midline, in the depression of the center of the suprasternal fossa.

Method First insert perpendicularly 0.2-0.3 cun and then direct the needle inferiorly along the posterior border of the manubrium of the sternum 0.5-1 cun.

Actions Bears counterflow Qi downward, benefits the throat and voice.

Indications Asthma, bronchitis, laryngopharyngitis, goiter, phrenospasm, neurogenic vomiting, esophageal spasm, and vocal fold disorders.

Stratified anatomy 1. skin; 2. subcutaneous tissue; 3. the point lies between the left and right sternocleidomastoid muscle tendons; 4. the point lies above the superior side of the suprasternal notch; 5. the point lies between the left and right sternothyroid muscles; 6. trachea.

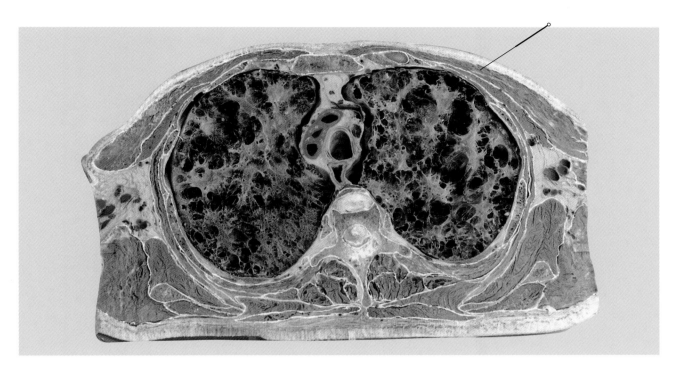

Fig. 4-2 (3) Transverse sectional figure of ST-14 Kufang

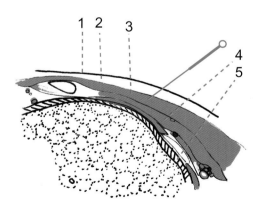

Transverse sectional figure
of ST-14 Kufang

ST-14 Kufang

Location In the 1st intercostal space, on the midline of the clavicle, 4 cun lateral to CV-20 Huagai.

Method Insert obliquely medially 0.3-0.4 cun.

Actions Bears counterflow Qi downward and opens the chest.

Indications Bronchitis and intercostal neuralgia.

Stratified anatomy 1. skin; 2. subcutaneous tissue; 3. pectoralis major muscle; 4. pectoralis minor muscle; 5. parietal pleura.

Cautions Do not insert too deeply or in the wrong direction to avoid injuring the tip of the axillary vein, or causing pneumothorax by piercing through the intercostal muscle, the parietal pleura, the pleural cavity, and the visceral pleura.

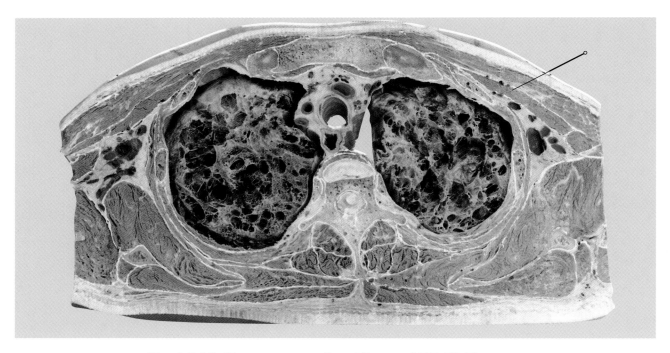

Fig. 4-2 (4) Transverse sectional figure of SP-20 Zhourong

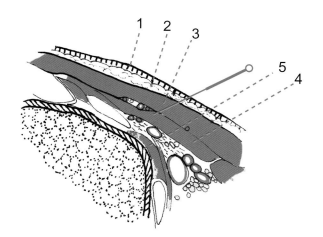

Transverse sectional figure
of SP-20 Zhourong (right)

SP-20 Zhourong

Location In the 2nd intercostal space, 6 cun lateral to the anterior midline.

Method Insert transversely or obliquely along the intercostal space 0.5 cun.

Actions Regulates Qi, bears Qi downward and opens the chest.

Indications Intercostal neuralgia, pleurisy, lung abscess, and bronchiectasis.

Stratified anatomy 1. skin; 2. subcutaneous tissue; 3. pectoralis major muscle; 4. pectoralis minor muscle; 5. parietal pleura.

Cautions Do not insert too deeply to avoid causing pneumothorax by piercing through the external and internal intercostal muscles, the parietal pleura, the pleural cavity, and the visceral pleura.

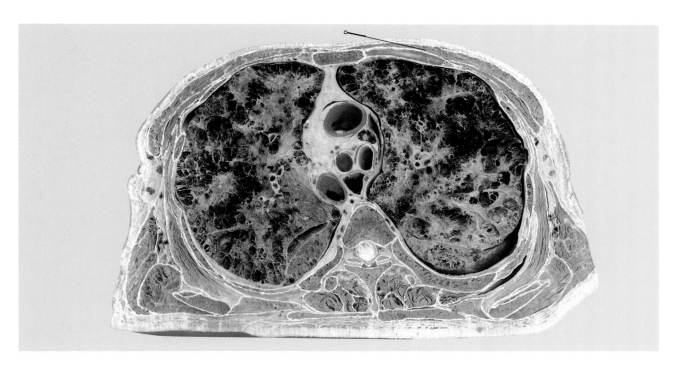

Fig. 4-2 (5) Transverse sectional figure of KI-25 Shencang

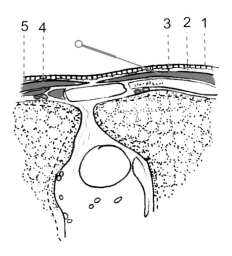

Transverse sectional figure
of KI-25 Shencang (right)

KI-25 Shencang

Location In the 2nd intercostal space, 2 cun lateral to CV-19 Zigong.

Method Insert transversely or obliquely toward the intercostal space 0.2-0.3 cun.

Actions Bears counterflow Lung and Stomach Qi downward.

Indications Bronchitis, vomiting and intercostal neuralgia.

Stratified anatomy 1. skin; 2. subcutaneous tissue; 3. pectoralis major muscle; 4. external intercostal tendon and internal intercostal muscle; 5. parietal pleura.

Cautions Do not insert too deeply to avoid causing pneumothorax by piercing through the parietal pleura, the pleural cavity and the visceral pleura.

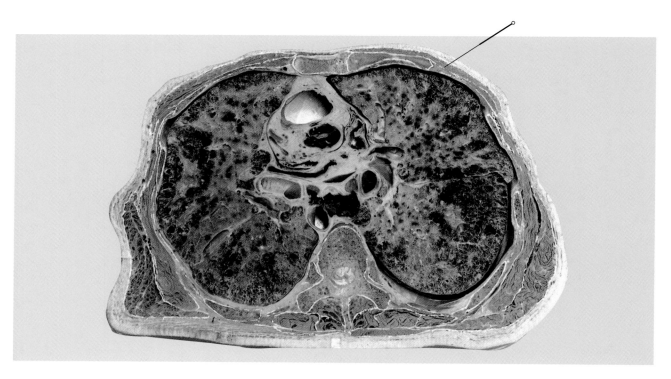

Fig. 4-2 (6) Transverse sectional figure of ST-16 Yingchuang

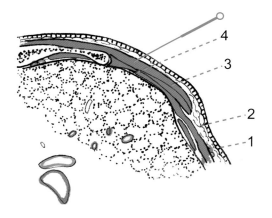

Transverse sectional figure
of ST-16 Yingchuang (right)

ST-16 Yingchuang

Location In the 3rd intercostal space, on the midline of the clavicle, 4 cun lateral to CV-18 Yutang.

Method Insert perpendicularly 0.2-0.3 cun or obliquely medially 0.3-0.5 cun.

Actions Stops coughing and benefits the breasts.

Indications Bronchitis, mastitis, asthma, intercostal neuralgia, borborygmi, and diarrhea.

Stratified anatomy 1. skin; 2. subcutaneous tissue; 3. pectoralis major muscle; 4. parietal pleura.

Cautions Do not insert too deeply to avoid causing pneumothorax by piercing through the internal and external intercostal muscles, the parietal pleura, the pleural cavity, and the visceral pleura.

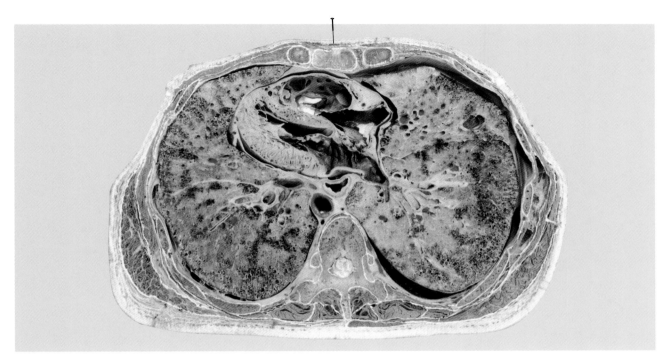

Fig. 4-2 (7) Transverse sectional figure of CV-17 Danzhong

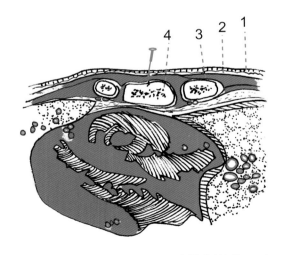

Transverse sectional figure of CV-17 Danzhong

CV-17 Danzhong

Location On the anterior midline 1.6 cun below CV-18 Yutang, on the midpoint of the line connecting the nipples.

Method Insert transversely inferiorly 0.5-1 cun.

Actions Regulates Qi, bears counterflow Lung and Stomach Qi downward, and benefits the breasts.

Indications Asthma, bronchitis, chest pain, mastitis, insufficient lactation, and intercostal neuralgia.

Stratified anatomy 1. skin; 2. subcutaneous tissue; 3. pectoralis major muscle; 4. body of sternum.

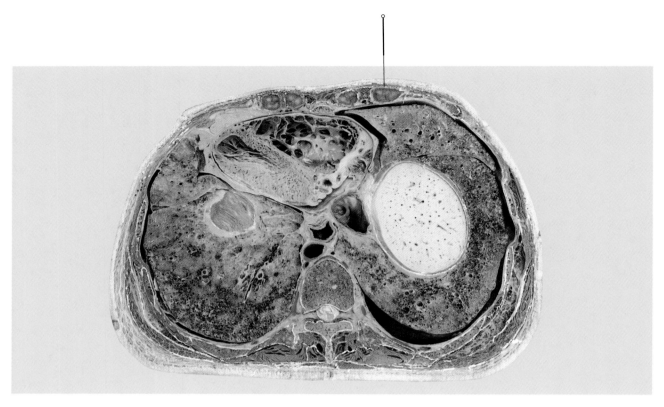

Fig. 4-2 (8) Transverse sectional figure of KI-22 Bulang

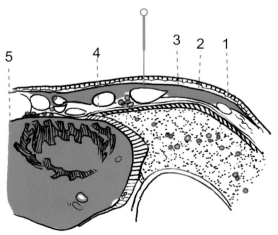

Transverse sectional figure of
KI-22 Bulang (right)

KI-22 Bulang

Location In the 5th intercostal space, 2 cun lateral to CV-16 Zhongting.

Method Insert perpendicularly or obliquely 0.3 cun.

Actions Opens the chest, bears Lung and Stomach Qi downward.

Indications Pleurisy, intercostal neuralgia, rhinitis, gastritis and bronchitis.

Stratified anatomy 1. skin; 2. subcutaneous tissue; 3. pectoralis major muscle; 4. parietal pleura; 5. pericardium.

Cautions Do not insert too deeply at right KI-22 Bulang to avoid causing pneumothorax by piercing through the external and internal intercostal muscles, the parietal pleura, the pleural cavity, and the visceral pleura and at left KI-22 Bulang to avoid injuring the left ventricle by piercing through the visceral pleura and the pericardium.

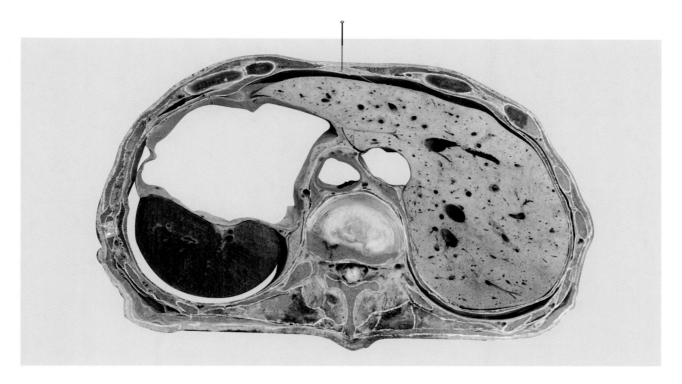

Fig. 4-2 (9) Transverse sectional figure of CV-15 Jiuwei

CV-15 Jiuwei

Location On the anterior midline of the upper abdomen, 1 cun distal to the sternocostal angle.

Method Insert obliquely inferiorly 0.5-1 cun.

Actions Regulates the Heart, bears Lung Qi downward and opens the chest.

Indications Angina pectoris, epilepsy, hiccup, schizophrenia, and asthma.

Stratified anatomy 1. skin; 2. subcutaneous tissue; 3. rectus abdominis muscle and sheath; 4. liver.

Cautions Do not insert too deeply perpendicularly, or the tip of the needle may pierce through the diaphragm, parietal peritoneum and subphrenic space of the peritoneal cavity. Needling deeper than 1.2 cun may injure the liver, and when combined with manipulations of lifting and thrusting and twirling, may cause serious damage.

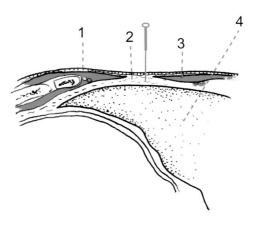

Transverse sectional figure
of CV-15 Jiuwei

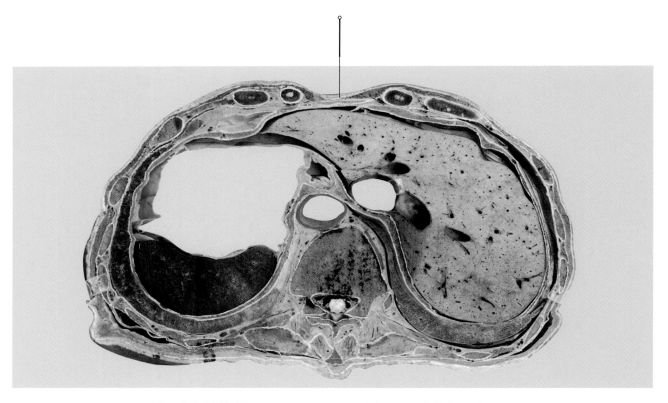

Fig. 4-2 (10) Transverse sectional figure of CV-14 Juque

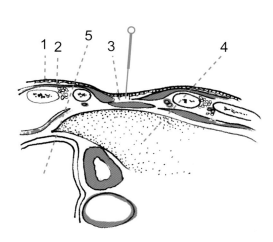

Transverse sectional figure
of CV-14 Juque

CV-14 Juque

Location On the anterior midline of the upper abdomen, 6 cun superior to the umbilicus.

Method Insert perpendicularly 0.5-1 cun.

Actions Bears Lung and Stomach Qi downward, calms the Spirit, regulates Heart Qi, and transforms Phlegm.

Indications Schizophrenia, epilepsy, angina pectoris, stomachache, vomiting, phreno-spasm, biliary ascariasis, and chronic hepatitis.

Stratified anatomy 1. skin; 2. subcutaneous tissue; 3. linea alba; 4. liver; 5. stomach.

Cautions Do not insert too deeply perpen-dicularly, or the tip of the needle may pierce through the intra-abdominal fascia, extra-peritoneal fat tissue, parietal peritoneum, and peritoneal cavity. Needling deeper than 1 cun may injure the liver and stomach, and when combined with manipulations of lifting and thrusting and twirling, may cause serious damage.

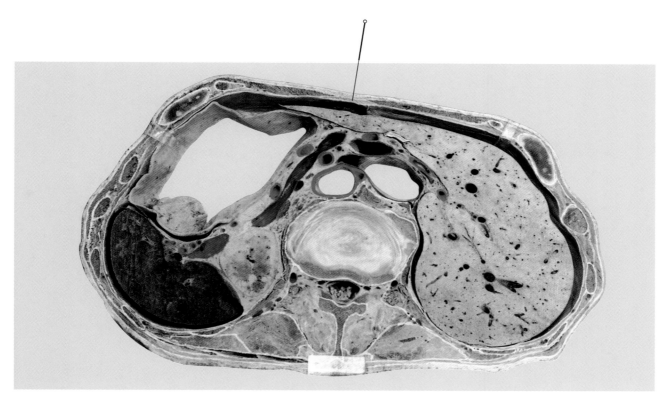

Fig. 4-2 (11) Transverse sectional figure of CV-13 Shangwan

CV-13 Shangwan

Location On the anterior midline of the upper abdomen, 5 cun superior to the umbilicus.

Method Insert perpendicularly 0.5-0.8 cun.

Actions Regulates the Heart and Stomach.

Indications Acute gastritis, gastrectasis, gastrospasm, and cardiospasm.

Stratified anatomy 1. skin; 2. subcutaneous tissue; 3. rectus abdominis muscle and sheath; 4. liver.

Cautions Do not insert too deeply perpendicularly, or the tip of the needle may pierce the parietal peritoneum and peritoneal cavity. Needling deeper than 1 cun may injure the left lobe of the liver, and when combined with manipulations of lifting and thrusting and twirling may cause serious damage .

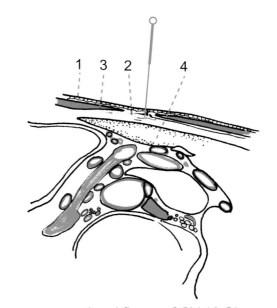

Transverse sectional figure of CV-13 Shangwan

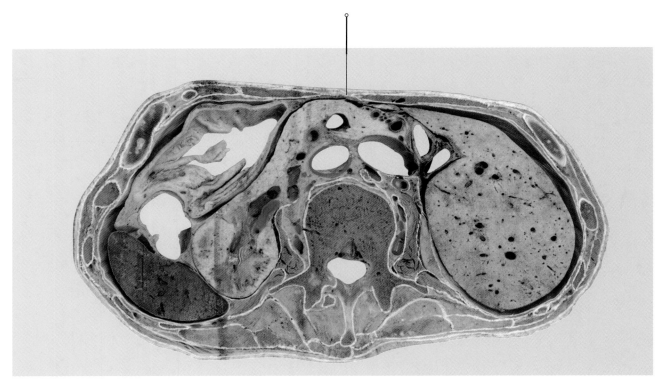

Fig. 4-2 (12) Transverse sectional figure of CV-12 Zhongwan

CV-12 Zhongwan

Location On the anterior midline of the upper abdomen, 4 cun superior to the umbilicus.

Method Insert perpendicularly 0.5-1 cun.

Actions Regulates Stomach Qi and bears counterflow Qi downward.

Indications Acute gastritis, chronic gastritis, gastric ulcer, gastroptosis, acute intestinal obstruction, stomachache, vomiting, abdominal distension, and diarrhea.

Stratified anatomy 1. skin; 2. subcutaneous tissue; 3. rectus abdominis muscle and sheath.

Cautions Do not insert too deeply perpendicularly, or the tip of the needle may pierce the parietal peritoneum and peritoneal cavity. Needling deeper than 1.5 cun may injure the gastric wall or bowel, and when combined with manipulations of lifting and thrusting and twirling may cause damage to the abdominal contents.

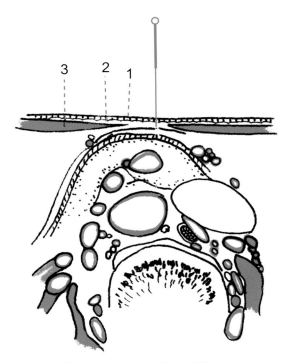

Transverse sectional figure
of CV-12 Zhongwan

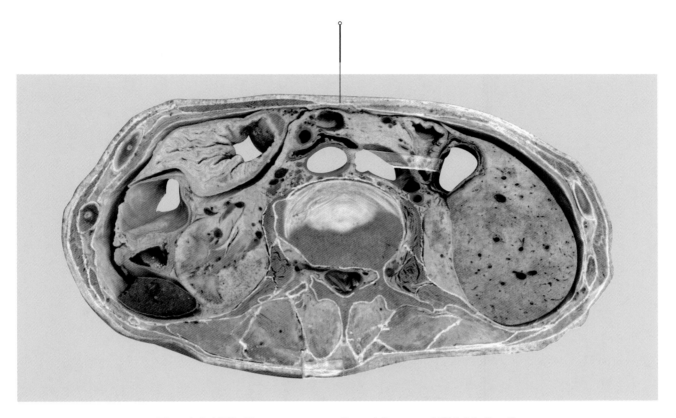

Fig. 4-2 (13) Transverse sectional figure of CV-11 Jianli

CV-11 Jianli

Location On the anterior midline of the upper abdomen, 3 cun superior to the umbilicus.
Method Insert perpendicularly 0.5-1 cun.
Actions Harmonizes the Middle Burner.
Indications Acute gastritis, chronic gastritis, angina pectoris, ascites, borborygmi, and abdominal pain.
Stratified anatomy 1. skin; 2. subcutaneous tissue; 3. rectus abdominis muscle and sheath.
Cautions Do not insert too deeply perpendicularly, or the tip of the needle may injure the transverse colon or the small intestine by piercing through the abdominal transverse fascia, the extraperitoneal fat tissue, the visceral peritoneum, and when combined with manipulations of lifting and thrusting and twirling, may cause serious damage.

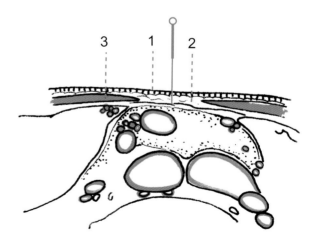

Transverse sectional figure of CV-11 Jianli

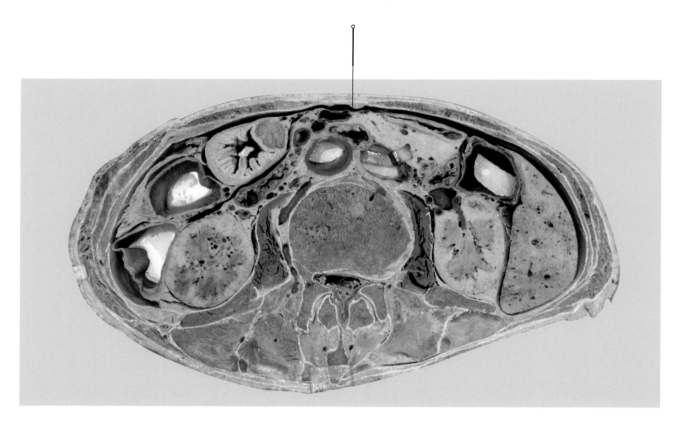

Fig. 4-2 (14) Transverse sectional figure of CV-10 Xiawan

CV-10 Xiawan

Location On the anterior midline of the upper abdomen, 2 cun superior to the umbilicus.

Method Insert perpendicularly 0.5-1 cun.

Actions Harmonizes the Stomach and regulates Qi.

Indications Dyspepsia, stomachache, gastroptosis, and diarrhea.

Stratified anatomy 1. skin; 2. subcutaneous tissue; 3. rectus abdominis muscle and sheath.

Cautions Do not insert too deeply perpendicularly, or the tip of the needle may injure the parietal peritoneum and peritoneal cavity. Needling deeper than 1 cun may injure the lower border of the stomach or the transverse colon, and when combined with manipulations of lifting and thrusting and twirling, may cause serious damage.

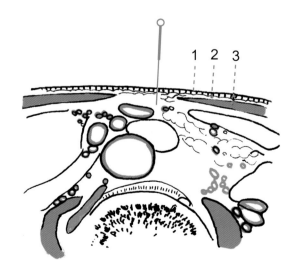

Transverse sectional figure of CV-10 Xiawan

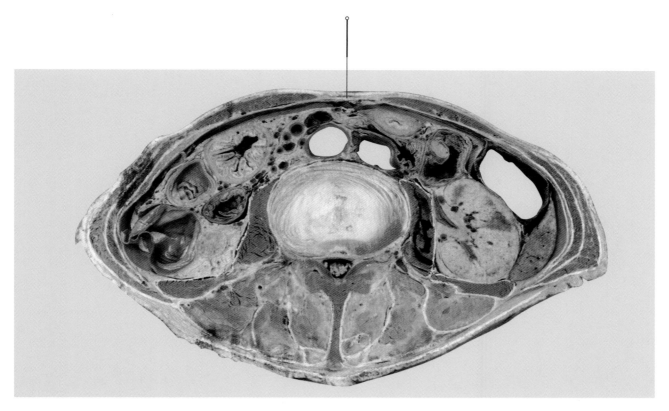

Fig. 4-2 (15) Transverse sectional figure of CV-9 Shuifen

CV-9 Shuifen

Location On the anterior midline of the upper abdomen, 1 cun superior to the umbilicus.

Method Insert perpendicularly 0.5-1 cun.

Actions Harmonizes Stomach Qi and dispels water accumulation.

Indications Ascites, vomiting, diarrhea, and nephritis.

Stratified anatomy 1. skin; 2. subcutaneous tissue; 3. rectus abdominis muscle and sheath.

Cautions Do not insert too deeply perpendicularly, or the tip of the needle may pierce the parietal peritoneum and peritoneal cavity. Needling deeper than 1 cun may injure the transverse colon, and when combined with manipulations of lifting and thrusting and twirling, may cause serious damage.

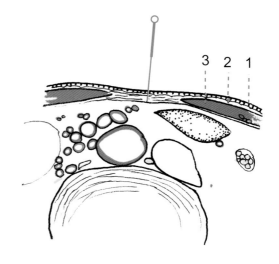

Transverse sectional figure of CV-9 Shuifen

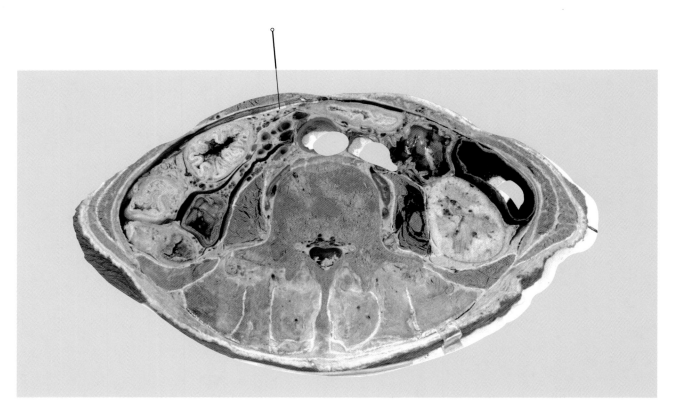

Fig. 4-2 (16) Transverse sectional figure of ST-25 Tianshu

ST-25 Tianshu

Location On the abdomen, 2 cun lateral to the umbilicus.

Method Insert perpendicularly 1-1.5 cun.

Actions: Regulates the Intestines, regulates Qi and Blood, and eliminates stagnation.

Indications Enteritis, bacillary dysentery, entero-paralysis, peritonitis, biliary ascariasis, endometrial infection, constipation, and abdominal pain.

Stratified anatomy 1. skin; 2. subcutaneous tissue; 3. rectus abdominis muscle and sheath.

Cautions Do not insert too deeply, or the tip of the needle may pierce the parietal peritoneum and peritoneal cavity. Needling deeper than 1.5 cun may injure the intestine, and when combined with manipulations of lifting and thrusting and twirling, may cause serious damage.

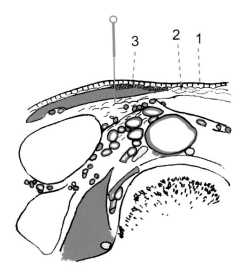

Transverse sectional figure
of ST-25 Tianshu (left)

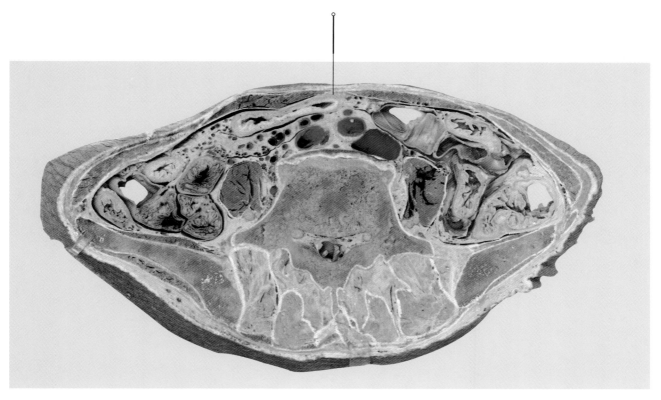

Fig. 4-2 (17) Transverse sectional figure of CV-7 Yinjiao

CV-7 Yinjiao

Location On the anterior midline of the lower abdomen, 1 cun distal to the umbilicus.

Method Insert perpendicularly 0.5 cun.

Actions Regulates menstruation and benefits the Lower Burner.

Indications Irregular menstruation, metrorrhagia and metrostaxis, leukorrhea, edema, pain due to hernia, and prolapse of the uterus.

Stratified anatomy 1. skin; 2. subcutaneous tissue; 3. rectus abdominis muscle and sheath.

Cautions Do not insert too deeply perpendicularly, or the tip of the needle may pierce the parietal peritoneum and peritoneal cavity. Needling deeper than 1 cun may injure the jejunum and ileum, with an even greater risk of damage when combined with lifting and thrusting and twirling manipulations.

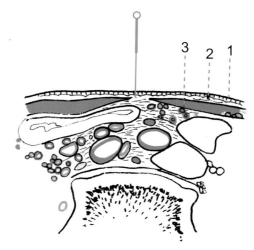

Transverse sectional figure of CV-7 Yinjiao

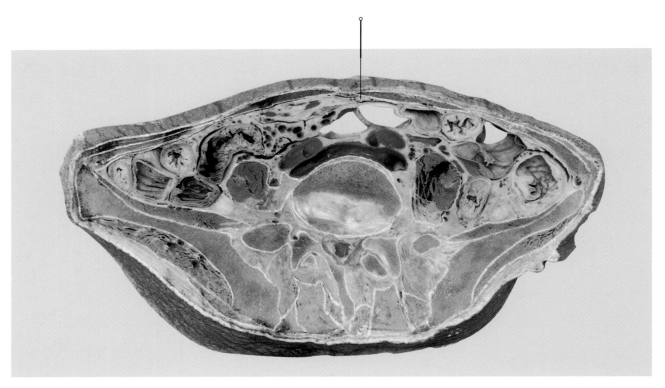

Fig. 4-2 (18) Transverse sectional figure of CV-6 Qihai

CV-6 Qihai

Location On the anterior midline of the lower abdomen, 1.5 cun distal to the umbilicus.

Method Insert perpendicularly 0.5-1 cun.

Actions Supplements the Kidneys and augments Qi, regulates Qi and Blood.

Indications Neurasthenia, abdominal distension, abdominal pain, irregular menstruation, dysmenor-rhea, enteroparalysis, enuresis, retention of urine, seminal emission, and impotence.

Stratified anatomy 1. skin; 2. subcutaneous tissue; 3. rectus abdominis muscle and sheath.

Cautions Do not insert too deeply perpendicularly, or the tip of the needle may pierce the parietal peritoneum and peritoneal cavity. Needling deeper than 1 cun may injure the jejunum and ileum. At over 2.5 cun in depth, the abdominal aorta may be injured, and there may be a greater risk of damage when using lifting and thrusting and twirling manipulations.

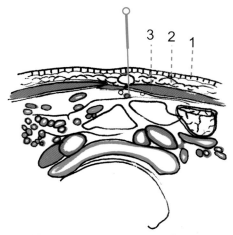

Transverse sectional figure
of CV-6 Qihai

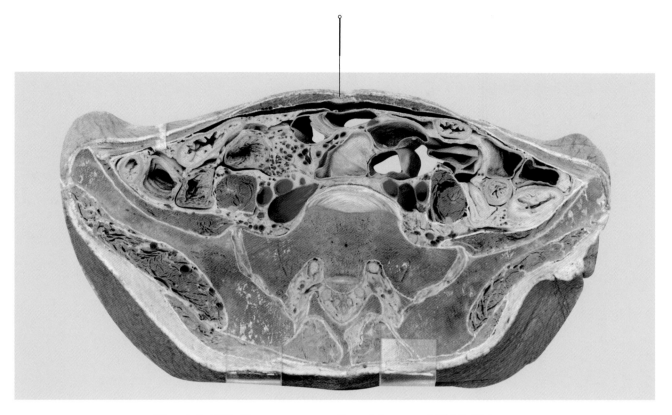

Fig. 4-2 (19) Transverse sectional figure of CV-5 Shimen

CV-5 Shimen

Location On the anterior midline of the lower abdomen, 2 cun distal to the umbilicus.

Method Insert perpendicularly 0.5-1 cun.

Actions Regulates Qi and Body Fluids, benefits the Uterus.

Indications Metrorrhagia and metrostaxis, amenorrhea, edema, retention of urine, and mastitis.

Stratified anatomy 1. skin; 2. subcutaneous tissue; 3. rectus abdominis muscle and sheath.

Cautions Do not insert too deeply perpendicularly, or the tip of the needle may pierce the intra-abdominal fascia, the extraperitoneal fat tissue, the parietal peritoneum, and the peritoneal cavity; if inserted further, it may injure the jejunum, with a greater risk of damage when using lifting and thrusting and twirling manipulations.

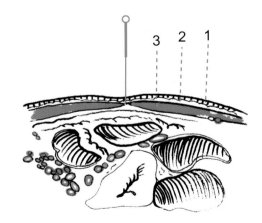

Transverse sectional figure
of CV-5 Shimen

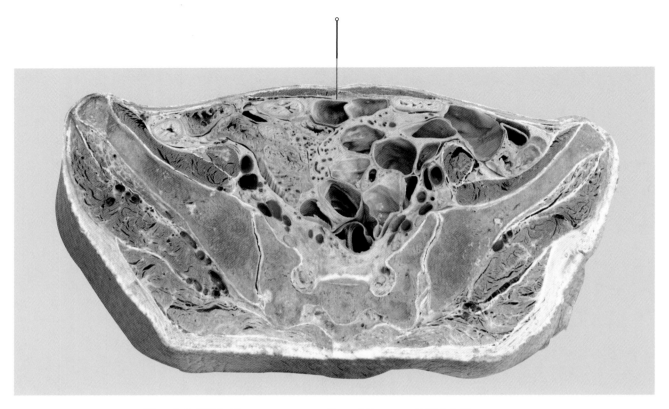

Fig. 4-2 (20) Transverse sectional figure of CV-4 Guanyuan

CV-4 Guanyuan

Location On the anterior midline of the lower abdomen, 3 cun distal to the umbilicus.

Method Insert perpendicularly 0.5-1 cun.

Actions Nourishes the Kidneys, regulates Qi and restores Yang.

Indications Abdominal pain, diarrhea, dysentery, urinary tract infection, nephritis, irregular menstruation, dysmenorrhea, leukorrhea, pelvic infection, dysfunctional uterine bleeding, prolapse of the uterus, seminal emission, impotence, and enuresis.

Stratified anatomy 1. skin; 2. subcutaneous tissue; 3. rectus abdominis muscle and sheath.

Cautions Do not insert too deeply perpendicularly, or the tip of the needle may injure the small intestine.

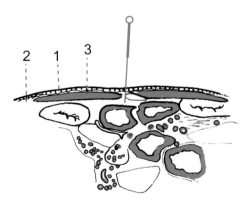

Transverse sectional figure
of CV-4 Guanyuan

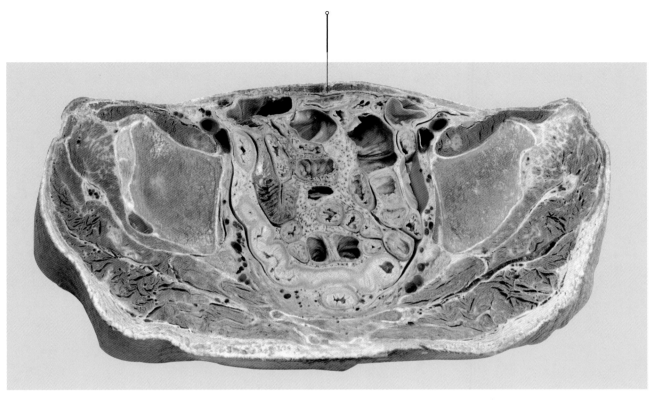

Fig. 4-2 (21) Transverse sectional figure of CV-3 Zhongji

CV-3 Zhongji

Location On the anterior midline of the lower abdomen, 4 cun distal to the umbilicus.

Method Insert perpendicularly 0.5-1 cun.

Actions Regulates the Uterus, clears Heat, dispels Dampness, and assists Qi transformation.

Indications Seminal emission, enuresis, frequent micturition, retention of urine, impotence, irregular menstruation, leukorrhea, sterility, nephritis, urinary tract infection, pelvic infection, dysmenorrhea, and sciatica.

Stratified anatomy 1. skin; 2. subcutaneous tissue; 3. rectus abdominis muscle and sheath.

Cautions Do not insert too deeply perpendicularly, or the tip of the needle may pierce the intra-abdominal fascia, the extraperitoneal fat tissue, the parietal peritoneum, and the peritoneal cavity; if inserted further, it may injure the ileum, with a greater risk of damage when using lifting and thrusting and twirling manipulations.

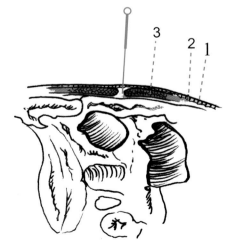

Transverse sectional figure of CV-3 Zhongji

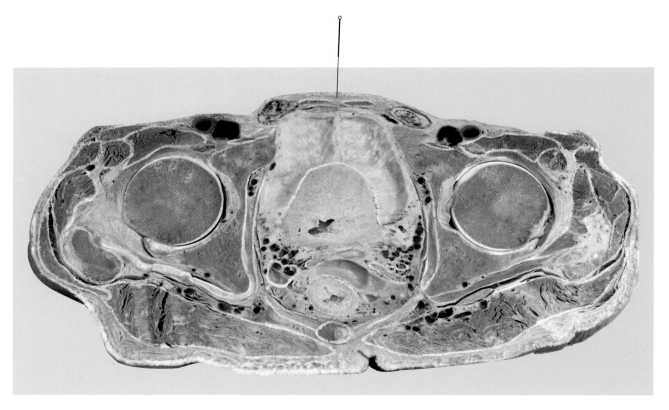

Fig. 4-2 (22) Transverse sectional figure of CV-2 Qugu

CV-2 Qugu

Location On the anterior midline of the lower abdomen, on the midpoint of the superior border of the pubic symphysis, 5 cun distal to the umbilicus.

Method Insert perpendicularly 0.5-1 cun.

Actions Regulates the Lower Burner and promotes urination.

Indications Irregular menstruation, prolapse of the uterus, cystitis, and constriction of the vulva.

Stratified anatomy 1. skin; 2. subcutaneous tissue; 3. pyramidalis muscle, rectus abdominis muscle and sheath.

Cautions Do not insert too deeply perpendicularly, or the tip of the needle may pierce the intra-abdominal fascia, the extraperitoneal fat tissue, the parietal peritoneum, and the peritoneal cavity; if inserted further, it may injure the ileum, with a greater risk of damage when using lifting and thrusting and twirling manipulations.

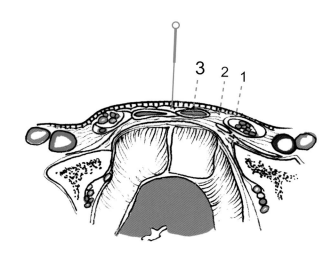

Transverse sectional figure
of CV-2 Qugu

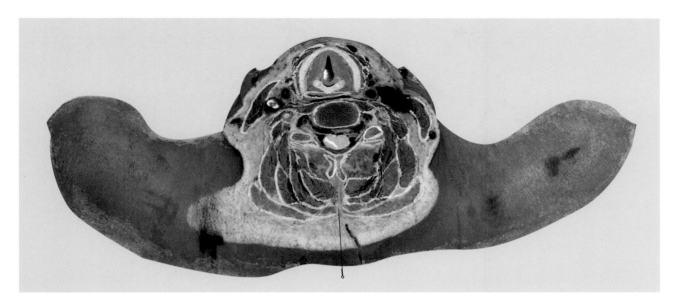

Fig. 4-2 (23) Transverse sectional figure of GV-14 Dazhui

GV-14 Dazhui

Location In the depression inferior to the spinous process of the 7th cervical vertebra.
Method Insert obliquely 0.5-0.8 cun.
Actions Expels Wind, consolidates the exterior, clears Heat, and calms the Spirit.
Indications Fever, sunstroke, epilepsy, schizophrenia, pulmonary tuberculosis, and sweating.
Stratified anatomy 1. skin; 2. subcutaneous tissue; 3. trapezius muscle; 4. supraspinous ligament; 5. interspinous ligament.
Cautions Do not insert too deeply, or the needle may pierce through the vertebral canal into the spinal cord with a greater risk of damage when combined with lifting and thrusting and twirling manipulations.

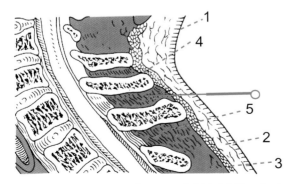

Sagittal sectional figure of GV-14 Dazhui

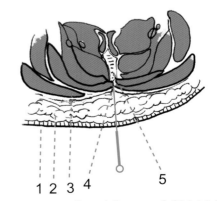

Transverse sectional figure of GV-14 Dazhui

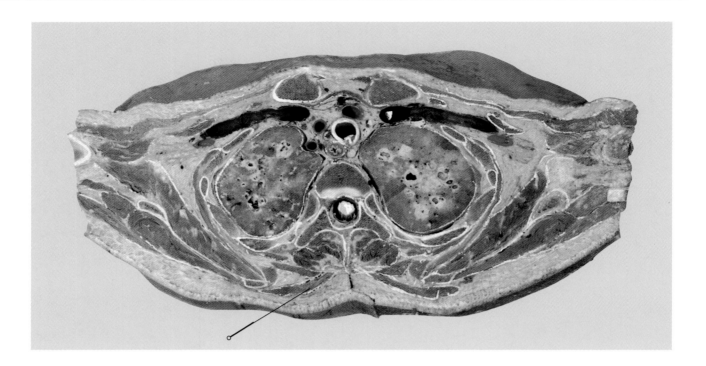

Fig. 4-2 (24) Transverse sectional figure of BL-13 Feishu

BL-13 Feishu

Location 1.5 cun lateral to the intervertebral space inferior to the spinous process of the 3rd thoracic vertebra.

Method Insert obliquely toward the spine 0.5 cun.

Actions Regulates Lung Qi, clears Heat and releases the exterior.

Indications Bronchitis, asthma, pneumonia, pulmonary tuberculosis, pleurisy, spontaneous sweating, and night sweating.

Stratified anatomy 1. skin; 2. subcutaneous tissue; 3. trapezius muscle; 4. rhomboid muscle; 5. sacrospinalis muscle.

Cautions Do not insert too deeply to avoid causing pneumothorax by piercing through the intercostal soft tissue, parietal pleura, pleural cavity, and visceral pleura.

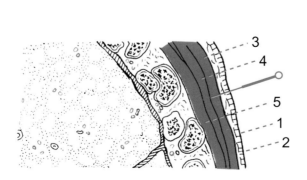

Sagittal sectional figure of BL-13 Feishu (left)

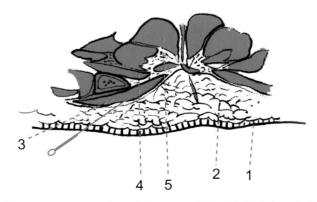

Transverse sectional figure of BL-13 Feishu (left)

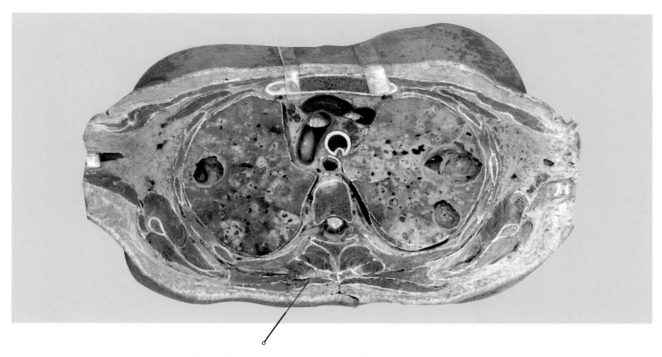

Fig. 4-2 (25) Transverse sectional figure of BL-14 Jueyinshu

BL-14 Jueyinshu

Location 1.5 cun lateral to the intervertebral space inferior to the spinous process of the 4th thoracic vertebra.

Method Insert obliquely 0.5-0.8 cun.

Actions Regulates Liver and Heart Qi and bears counterflow Qi downward.

Indications Rheumatic heart disease, neurasthenia and intercostal neuralgia.

Stratified anatomy 1. skin; 2. subcutaneous tissue; 3. trapezius muscle; 4. rhomboid muscle; 5. sacrospinalis muscle; 6. parietal pleura.

Cautions Do not insert too deeply to avoid causing pneumothorax by piercing through the intercostal soft tissue, parietal

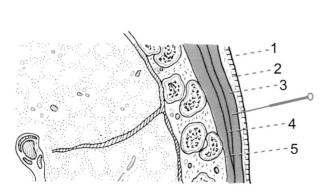

Sagittal sectional figure
of BL-14 Jueyinshu (left)

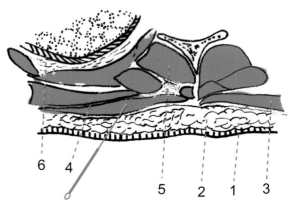

Transverse sectional figure
of BL-14 Jueyinshu (left)

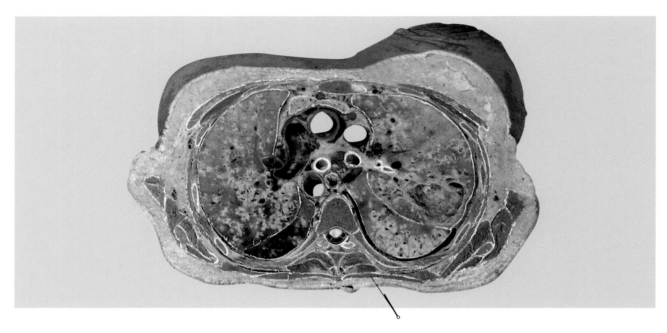

Fig. 4-2 (26) Transverse sectional figure of BL-15 Xinshu

BL-15 Xinshu

Location 1.5 cun lateral to the intervertebral space inferior to the spinous process of the 5th thoracic vertebra.

Method Insert obliquely 0.5 cun.

Actions Regulates Qi and Blood, calms the Heart and Spirit.

Indications Neurasthenia, intercostal neuralgia, rheumatic heart disease, atrial fibrillation, tachycardia, schizophrenia, epilepsy, and anxiety disorder.

Stratified anatomy 1. skin; 2. subcutaneous tissue; 3. trapezius muscle; 4. sacrospinalis muscle; 5. parietal pleura.

Cautions Do not insert too deeply to avoid causing pneumothorax by piercing through the intercostal soft tissue, parietal pleura, pleural cavity, and visceral pleura.

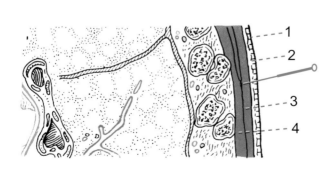

Sagittal sectional figure
of BL-15 Xinshu (right)

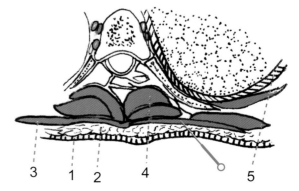

Transverse sectional figure
of BL-15 Xinshu (right)

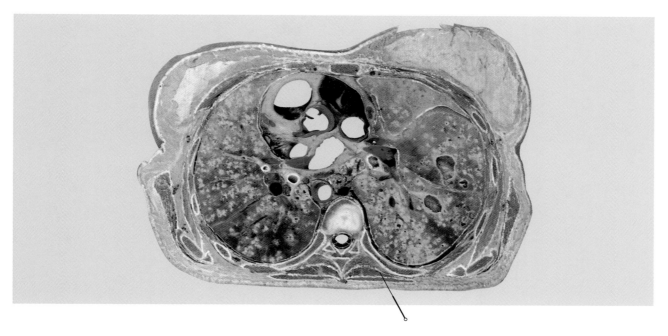

Fig. 4-2 (27) Transverse sectional figure of BL-16 Dushu

BL-16 Dushu

Location 1.5 cun lateral to the intervertebral space inferior to the spinous process of the 6th thoracic vertebra.

Method Insert obliquely 0.5 cun.

Actions Regulates Qi in the chest and bears counterflow Qi downward.

Indications Endocarditis, epicarditis, abdominal pain, borborygmi, phrenospasm, mastitis, pruritus, and psoriasis.

Stratified anatomy 1. skin; 2. subcutaneous tissue; 3. trapezius muscle; 4. sacrospinalis muscle; 5. parietal pleura.

Cautions Do not insert too deeply to avoid causing pneumothorax by piercing through the intercostal soft tissue, parietal pleura, pleural cavity, and visceral pleura.

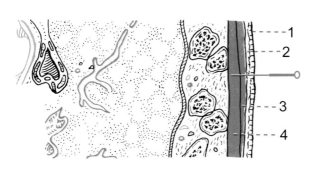

Sagittal sectional figure
of BL-16 Dushu (right)

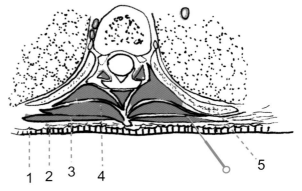

Transverse sectional figure
of BL-16 Dushu (right)

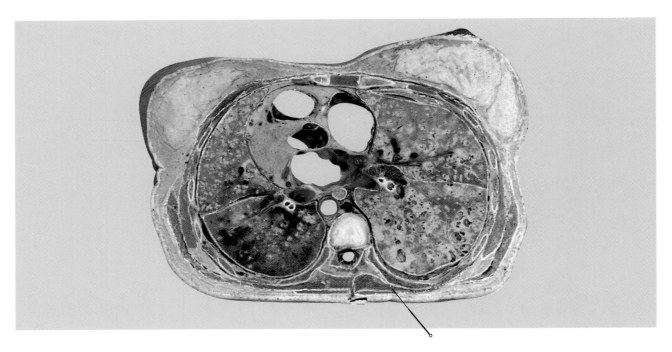

Fig. 4-2 (28) Transverse sectional figure of BL-17 Geshu

BL-17 Geshu

Location 1.5 cun lateral to the intervertebral space inferior to the spinous process of the 7th thoracic vertebra.

Method Insert obliquely 0.5 cun.

Actions Regulates the Blood, transforms Blood stasis, opens the chest, and strengthens Deficiency.

Indications Anemia, chronic bleeding, phrenospasm, vomiting, urticaria, lymphoid tuberculosis, and esophageal stricture.

Stratified anatomy 1. skin; 2. subcutaneous tissue; 3. trapezius muscle; 4. latissimus dorsi muscle; 5. sacrospinalis muscle; 6. parietal pleura.

Cautions Do not insert too deeply to avoid causing pneumothorax by piercing through the intercostal soft tissue, parietal pleura, pleural cavity, and visceral pleura.

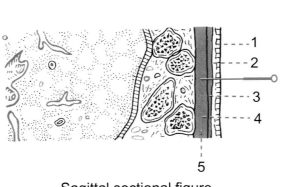

Sagittal sectional figure
of BL-17 Geshu (right)

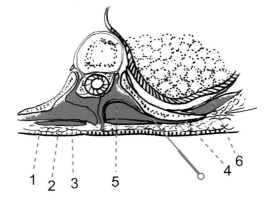

Transverse sectional figure
of BL-17 Geshu (right)

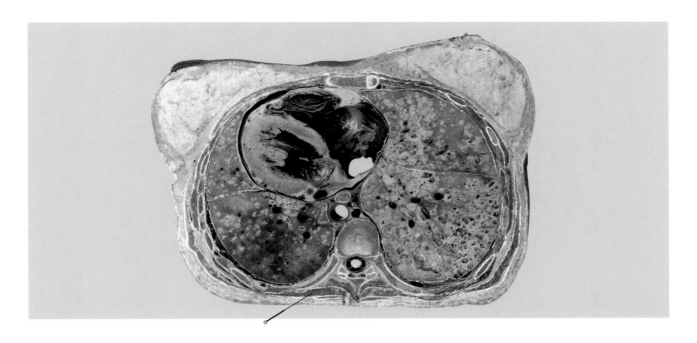

Fig. 4-2 (29) Transverse sectional figure of EX-B-3 Weiwanxiashu

EX-B-3 Weiwanxiashu (also called Weiguanxiashu)

Location 1.5 cun lateral to the intervertebral space inferior to the spinous process of the 8th thoracic vertebra.

Method Insert obliquely 0.5 cun.

Actions Regulates Qi, bears counterflow Qi downward, clears Heat, and generates Body Fluids.

Indications Stomachache, pancreatitis, vomiting, pain in the chest and hypochondrium, cough, and dry throat.

Stratified anatomy 1. skin; 2. subcutaneous tissue; 3. trapezius muscle; 4. latissimus dorsi muscle; 5. sacrospinalis muscle; 6. parietal pleura.

Cautions Do not insert too deeply to avoid causing pneumothorax by piercing through the intercostal soft tissue, parietal pleura, pleural cavity, and visceral pleura.

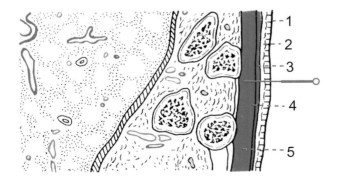

Sagittal sectional figure
of EX-B-3 Weiwanxiashu (left)

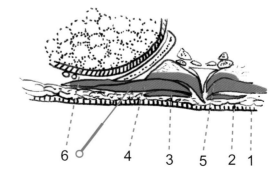

Transverse sectional figure
of EX-B-3 Weiwanxiashu (left)

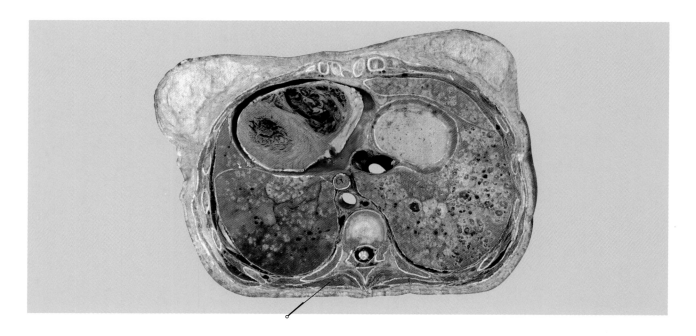

Fig. 4-2 (30) Transverse sectional figure of BL-18 Ganshu

BL-18 Ganshu

Location 1.5 cun lateral to the intervertebral space inferior to the spinous process of the 9th thoracic vertebra.

Method Insert obliquely 0.5 cun.

Actions Regulates Liver Qi, nourishes Liver Blood, cools Fire, and extinguishes Wind.

Indications Hepatitis, cholecystitis, stomachache, eye disorders, intercostal neuralgia, neurasthenia, and irregular menstruation.

Stratified anatomy 1. skin; 2. subcutaneous tissue; 3. trapezius muscle; 4. latissimus dorsi muscle; 5. sacrospinalis muscle; 6. parietal pleura.

Cautions Do not insert too deeply to avoid causing pneumothorax by piercing through the intercostal soft tissue, parietal pleura, pleural cavity, and visceral pleura.

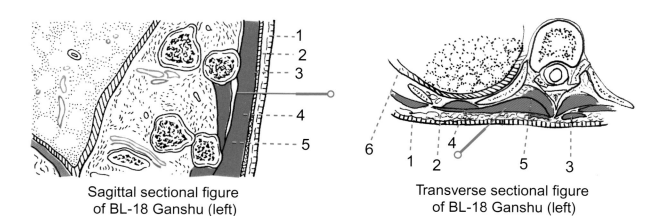

Sagittal sectional figure
of BL-18 Ganshu (left)

Transverse sectional figure
of BL-18 Ganshu (left)

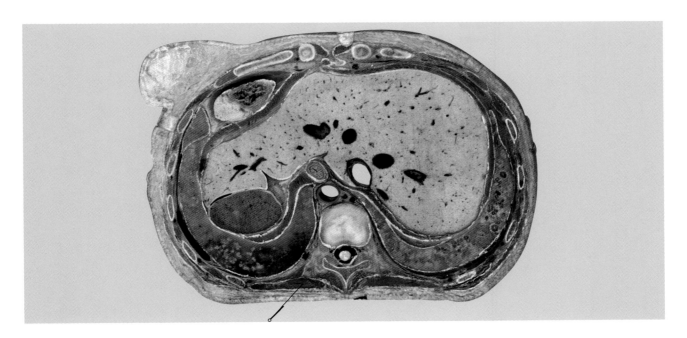

Fig. 4-2 (31) Transverse sectional figure of BL-19 Danshu

BL-19 Danshu

Location 1.5 cun lateral to the intervertebral space inferior to the spinous process of the 10th thoracic vertebra.

Method Insert obliquely 0.5 cun.

Actions Clears Damp-Heat from the Liver and Gallbladder, regulates Qi and calms the Stomach.

Indications Hepatitis, cholecystitis, stomachache, biliary ascariasis, lymphoid tuberculosis, abdominal distension, and pain in the chest and hypochondrium.

Stratified anatomy 1. skin; 2. subcutaneous tissue; 3. trapezius muscle; 4. latissimus dorsi muscle; 5. sacrospinalis muscle; 6. parietal pleura.

Cautions Do not insert too deeply to avoid causing pneumothorax by piercing through the intercostal soft tissue, parietal pleura, pleural cavity, and visceral pleura.

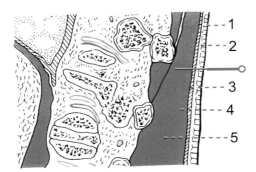

Sagittal sectional figure
of BL-19 Danshu (left)

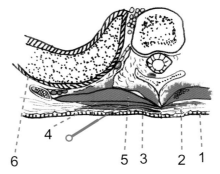

Transverse sectional figure
of BL-19 Danshu (left)

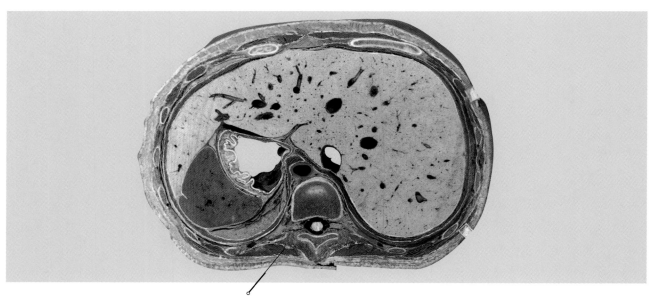

Fig. 4-2 (32) Transverse sectional figure of BL-20 Pishu

BL-20 Pishu

Location 1.5 cun lateral to the intervertebral space inferior to the spinous process of the 11th thoracic vertebra.

Method Insert obliquely 0.5 cun.

Actions Supplements Spleen Qi, transforms Dampness, and harmonizes Qi and Blood.

Indications Gastritis, ulcers of the upper gastrointestinal tract, gastroptosis, neurogenic vomiting, dyspepsia, hepatitis, enteritis, edema, anemia, hepatosplenomegaly, chronic bleeding, prolapse of the uterus, urticaria, and weakness of the extremities.

Stratified anatomy 1. skin; 2. subcutaneous tissue; 3. trapezius muscle; 4. latissimus dorsi muscle; 5. sacrospinalis muscle; 6. parietal pleura.

Cautions Do not insert too deeply to avoid causing pneumothorax by piercing through the intercostal soft tissue, parietal pleura, pleural cavity, and visceral pleura.

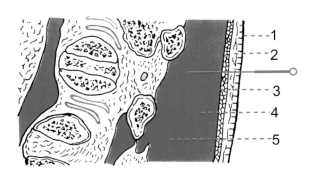

Sagittal sectional figure
of BL-20 Pishu (left)

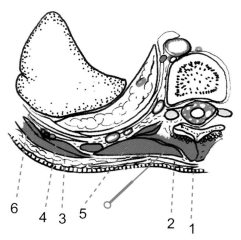

Transverse sectional figure
of BL-20 Pishu (left)

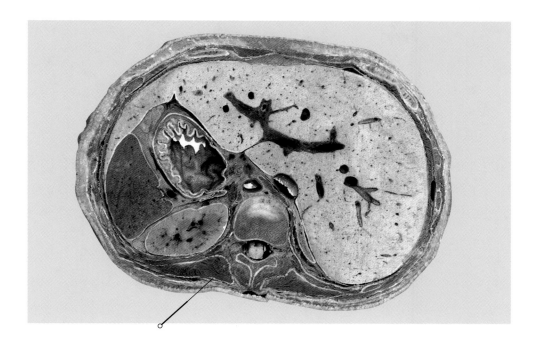

Fig. 4-2 (33) Transverse sectional figure of BL-21 Weishu

BL-21 Weishu

Location 1.5 cun lateral to the intervertebral space inferior to the spinous process of the 12th thoracic vertebra.

Method Insert obliquely 0.5 cun.

Actions Regulates the Stomach, transforms Dampness and harmonizes the Middle Burner.

Indications Stomachache, gastritis, gastrectasis, gastroptosis, ulcers of the upper gastrointestinal tract, pancreatitis, hepatitis, enteritis, anorexia, insomnia, and spinal pain.

Stratified anatomy 1. skin; 2. subcutaneous tissue; 3. thoracolumbar fascia and aponeurosis of the latissimus dorsi muscle; 4. sacrospinalis muscle; 5. kidney; 6. liver.

Cautions Do not insert too deeply to avoid injuring the liver and kidneys.

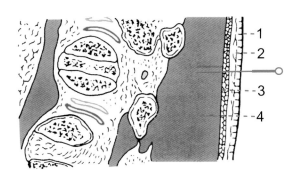

Sagittal sectional figure
of BL-21 Weishu (left)

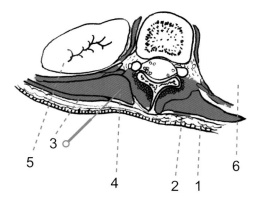

Transverse sectional figure
of BL-21 Weishu (left)

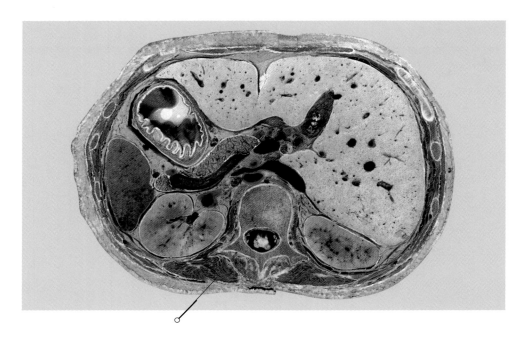

Fig. 4-2 (34) Transverse sectional figure of BL-22 Sanjiaoshu

BL-22 Sanjiaoshu

Location 1.5 cun lateral to the intervertebral space inferior to the spinous process of the 1st lumbar vertebra.

Method Insert obliquely medially 1-2 cun.

Actions Eliminates Dampness, promotes urination, and regulates the Triple Burner, Spleen and Stomach.

Indications Gastritis, enteritis, nephritis, ascites, retention of urine, enuresis, neurasthenia, and lumbago.

Stratified anatomy 1. skin; 2. subcutaneous tissue; 3. thoracolumbar fascia and aponeurosis of the latissimus dorsi muscle; 4. sacrospinalis muscle; 5. kidney.

Cautions Do not insert too deeply to avoid injuring the kidneys and liver (on the right side).

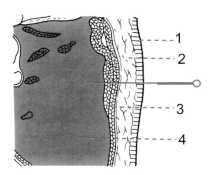

Sagittal sectional figure
of BL-22 Sanjiaoshu (left)

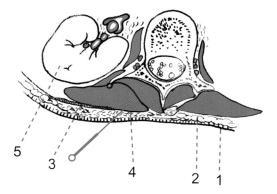

Transverse sectional figure
of BL-22 Sanjiaoshu (left)

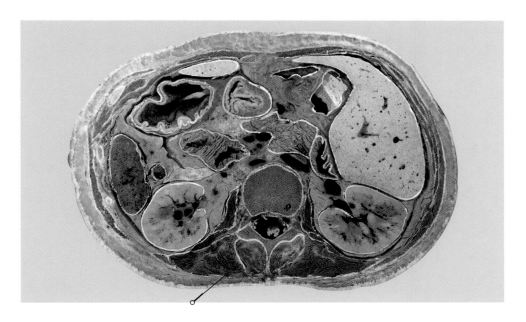

Fig. 4-2 (35) Transverse sectional figure of BL-23 Shenshu

BL-23 Shenshu

Location 1.5 cun lateral to the intervertebral space inferior to the spinous process of the 2nd lumbar vertebra.

Method Insert obliquely medially 1-2 cun.

Actions Supplements Kidney Yin, Qi and Yang, strengthens the lumbar vertebrae, and benefits the ears and eyes.

Indications Nephritis, renal colic, nephroptosis, lumbago, seminal emission, enuresis, impotence, irregular menstruation, asthma, tinnitus, deafness, anemia, lumbar soft tissue injury, and poliomyelitis sequelae.

Stratified anatomy 1. skin; 2. subcutaneous tissue; 3. thoracolumbar fascia and aponeurosis of the latissimus dorsi muscle; 4. sacrospinalis muscle; 5. kidney.

Cautions Do not insert too deeply to avoid injuring the kidneys.

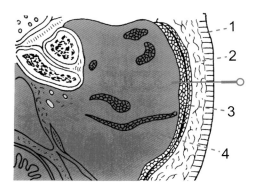

Sagittal sectional figure
of BL-23 Shenshu (left)

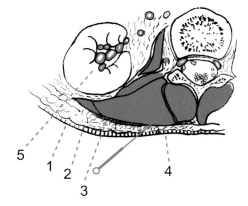

Transverse sectional figure
of BL-23 Shenshu (left)

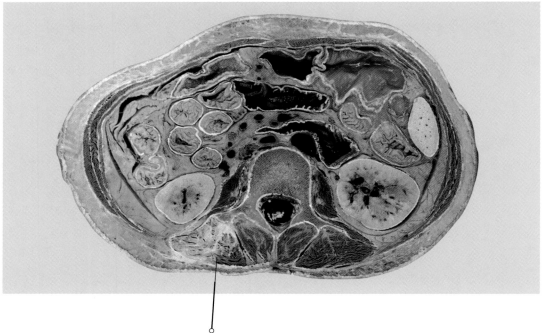

Fig. 4-2 (36) Transverse sectional figure of BL-24 Qihaishu

BL-24 Qihaishu

Location 1.5 cun lateral to the intervertebral space inferior to the spinous process of the 3rd lumbar vertebra.

Method Insert perpendicularly 1-2 cun.

Actions Regulates Qi and Blood, strengthens the lower back and knees.

Indications Lumbago, spinal pain, hemorrhoids, irregular menstruation, dysfunctional uterine bleeding, and paralysis of the lower extremities.

Stratified anatomy 1. skin; 2. subcutaneous tissue; 3. thoracolumbar fascia and aponeurosis of the latissimus dorsi muscle; 4. sacrospinalis muscle.

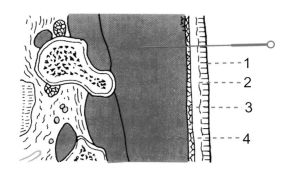

Sagittal sectional figure
of BL-24 Qihaishu (left)

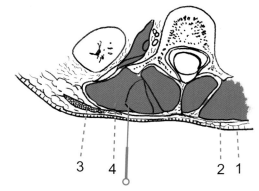

Transverse sectional figure
of BL-24 Qihaishu (left)

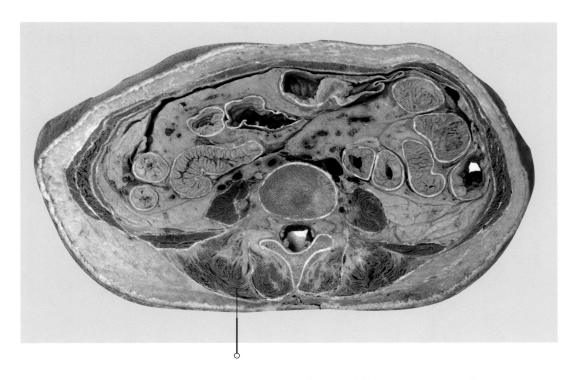

Fig. 4-2 (37) Transverse sectional figure of BL-25 Dachangshu

BL-25 Dachangshu

Location 1.5 cun lateral to the intervertebral space inferior to the spinous process of the 4th lumbar vertebra.

Method Insert perpendicularly 1-2 cun or insert obliquely laterally 2-3 cun.

Actions Regulates the Intestines and benefits the lower back and knees.

Indications Pain in the waist and lower extremities, lumbar sprain, sacroiliac arthralgia, enteritis, dysentery, and constipation.

Stratified anatomy 1. skin; 2. subcutaneous tissue; 3. thoracolumbar fascia; 4. sacrospinalis muscle.

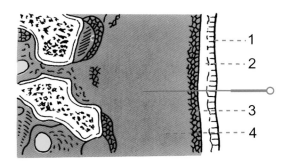

Sagittal sectional figure
of BL-25 Dachangshu (left)

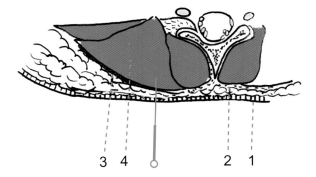

Transverse sectional figure
of BL-25 Dachangshu (left)

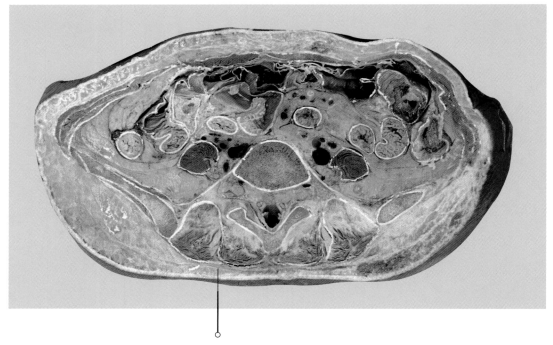

Fig. 4-2 (38) Transverse sectional figure of BL-26 Guanyuanshu

BL-26 Guanyuanshu

Location 1.5 cun lateral to the intervertebral space inferior to the spinous process of the 5th lumbar vertebra.

Method Insert perpendicularly 1-2 cun or insert obliquely laterally 2-3 cun.

Actions Regulates the Lower Burner and strengthens the lower back and knees.

Indications Chronic enteritis, lumbago, diabetes, anemia, chronic pelvic infection, and cystitis.

Stratified anatomy 1. skin; 2. subcutaneous tissue; 3. thoracolumbar fascia; 4. sacrospinalis muscle.

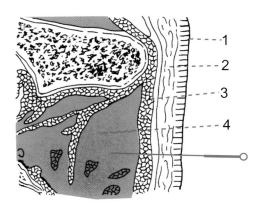

Sagittal sectional figure
of BL-26 Guanyuanshu (left)

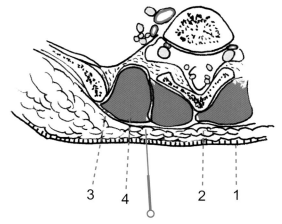

Transverse sectional figure
of BL-26 Guanyuanshu (left)

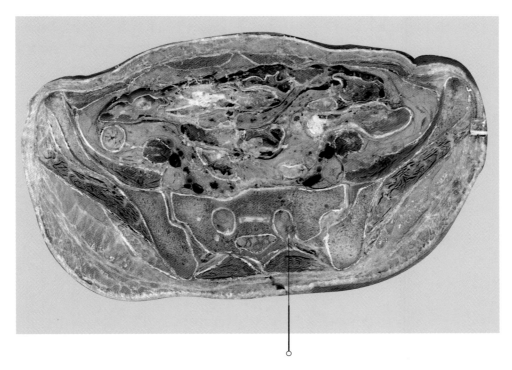

Fig. 4-2 (39) Transverse sectional figure of BL-31Shangliao

BL-31 Shangliao

Location On the sacrum, 1 cun lateral to the intervertebral space inferior to the spinous process of the 1st sacral vertebra, over the 1st posterior sacral foramen.

Method Insert perpendicularly 1-2 cun.

Actions Regulates the Lower Burner and benefits the lower back and legs.

Indications Diseases of the lumbosacral articulation, sciatica, irregular menstruation, difficult labor, leukorrhea, pelvic infection, orchitis, paralysis of the lower extremities, and poliomyelitis.

Stratified anatomy 1. skin; 2. subcutaneous tissue; 3. superficial layer of the thoracolumbar fascia; 4. sacrospinalis muscle; 5. 1st sacral nerve.

Cautions At over 1.2 cun in depth, the tip of the needle may pierce through the 1st posterior sacral foramen, and then the posterior branches of the 1st sacral nerve and 1st sacral nerve trunk, resulting in an intense electric shock-like sensation radiating toward the legs.

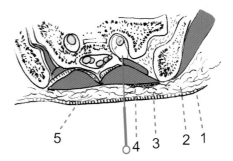

Transverse sectional figure
of BL-31 Shangliao (right)

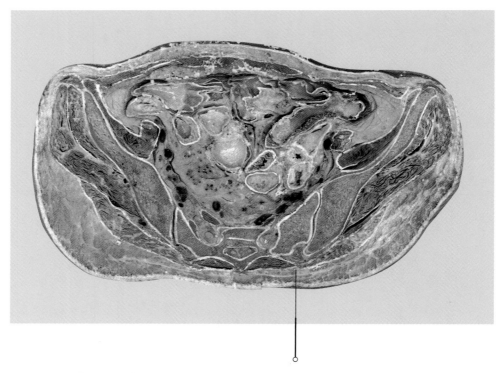

Fig. 4-2 (40) Transverse sectional figure of BL-32 Ciliao

BL-32 Ciliao

Location On the sacrum, 1 cun lateral to the intervertebral space inferior to the spinous process of the 2nd sacral vertebra, over the 2nd posterior sacral foramen.

Method Insert perpendicularly 1-2 cun.

Actions Regulates the Lower Burner, benefits the lower back and legs, regulates menstruation, and stops vaginal discharge.

Indications Diseases of the lumbosacral articulation, sciatica, irregular menstruation, difficult labor, leukorrhea, pelvic infection, orchitis, paralysis of the lower extremities, and poliomyelitis.

Stratified anatomy 1. skin; 2. subcutaneous tissue; 3. superficial layer of the thoracolumbar fascia; 4. sacrospinalis muscle.

Cautions At over 1.2 cun in depth, the tip of the needle may pierce through the 2nd posterior sacral foramen, and then the posterior branches of the 2nd sacral nerve and 2nd sacral nerve trunk, resulting in an intense electric shock-like sensation radiating toward the legs and genitalia.

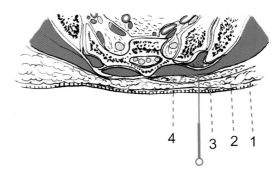

Transverse sectional figure
of BL-32 Ciliao (right)

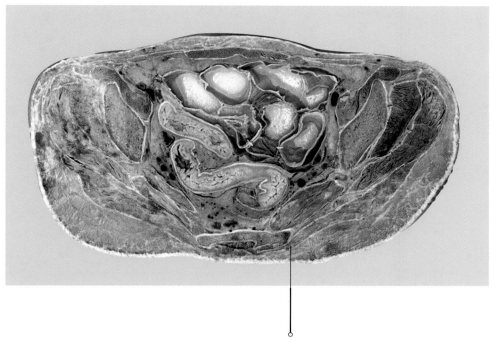

Fig. 4-2 (41) Transverse sectional figure of BL-33 Zhongliao

BL-33 Zhongliao

Location On the sacrum, 1 cun lateral to the intervertebral space inferior to the spinous process of the 3rd sacral vertebra, over the 3rd posterior sacral foramen.

Method Insert perpendicularly 1-2 cun.

Actions Regulates the Lower Burner, benefits the lower back and legs, promotes urination, and regulates menstruation.

Indications Diseases of the lumbosacral articulation, sciatica, irregular menstruation, difficult labor, leukorrhea, pelvic infection, orchitis, paralysis of the lower extremities, and poliomyelitis.

Stratified anatomy 1. skin; 2. subcutaneous tissue; 3. internal border of the gluteus maximus muscle; 4. superficial layer of the thoracolumbar fascia; 5. origin of the sacrospinalis muscle.

Cautions At over 1.2 cun in depth, the tip of the needle may pierce through the 3rd posterior sacral foramen, and then the posterior branches of the 3rd sacral nerve and 3rd sacral nerve trunk, resulting in an intense electric shock-like sensation radiating toward the buttocks and genitalia.

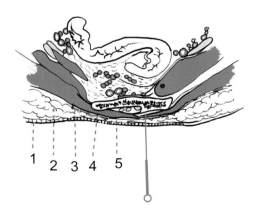

Transverse sectional figure
of BL-33 Zhongliao (right)

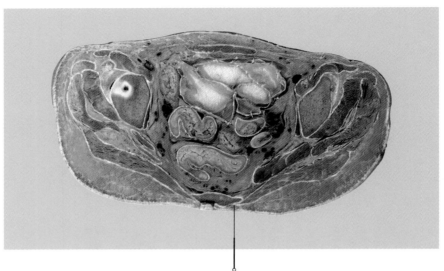

Fig. 4-2 (42) Transverse sectional figure of BL-34 Xialiao

BL-34 Xialiao

Location On the sacrum, 1 cun lateral to the intervertebral space inferior to the spinous process of the 4th sacral vertebra, over the 4th posterior sacral foramen.

Method Insert perpendicularly 1-2 cun.

Actions Regulates menstruation, stops vaginal discharge, and benefits the lower back and legs.

Indications Diseases of the lumbosacral articulation, sciatica, irregular menstruation, difficult labor, leukorrhea, pelvic infection, orchitis, paralysis of the lower extremities, and poliomyelitis.

Stratified anatomy 1. skin; 2. subcutaneous tissue; 3. internal border of the gluteus maximus muscle; 4. superficial layer of thoracolumbar fascia; 5. origin of the sacrospinalis muscle.

Cautions At over 1.2 cun in depth, the tip of the needle may pierce through the 4th posterior sacral foramen, and then the posterior branches of the 4th sacral nerve and 4th sacral nerve trunk, resulting in an intense electric shock-like sensation radiating toward the anus.

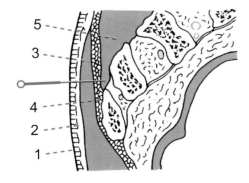

Sagittal sectional figure
of BL-34 Xialiao

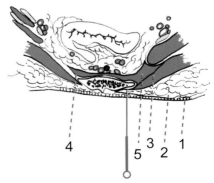

Transverse sectional figure
of BL-34 Xialiao (right)

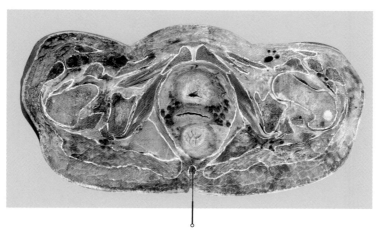

Fig. 4-2 (43) Transverse sectional figure of GV-1 Changqiang

GV-1 Changqiang

Location Inferior to the tip of the coccyx, at the midpoint of the line connecting the tip of the coccyx and the anus.

Method Insert obliquely 0.5-1 cun, the tip of needle pierces upward parallel to the coccyx and sacrum.

Actions Frees the channels, regulates the Intestines and calms the Spirit.

Indications Hemorrhoids, proctoptosis, eczema of the scrotum, diarrhea, impotence, and schizophrenia.

Stratified anatomy 1. skin; 2. subcutaneous tissue; 3. sacrotuberous ligament; 4. levator ani muscle; 5. rectum.

Cautions Do not insert too deeply, as the tip of the needle may pierce the rectum, and, when combined with manipulations of lifting and thrusting and twirling, may result in a fecal fistula when abdominal pressure increases during defecation. Deep infection may result in pelvic peritonitis while superficial infection may lead to ischiorectal abscess.

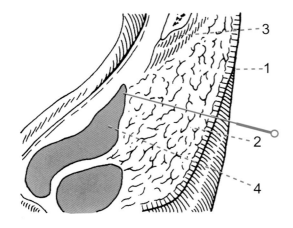

Sagittal sectional figure
of GV-1 Changqiang

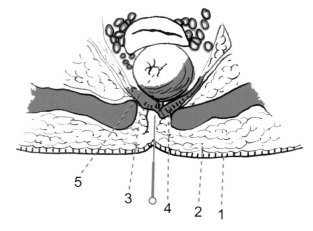

Transverse sectional figure
of GV-1 Changqiang

5 Sectional figures of acupuncture points on the limbs

ACUPUNCTURE POINTS ON THE ARM AND HAND

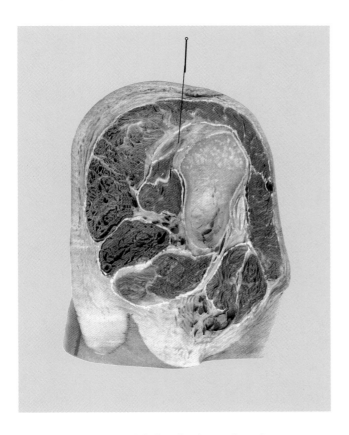

Fig. 5-1 (1) Sagittal sectional figure of LI-15 Jianyu (left)

LI-15 Jianyu

Location On the midpoint of the proximal part of the deltoid muscle, between the acromion and the greater tuberosity of the humerus.

Method Insert perpendicularly 0.8 cun.

Actions Expels Wind-Damp, benefits the shoulders, eliminates Wind, and regulates Qi and Blood.

Indications Hemiplegia, hypertension, pain in the shoulder joint, scapulohumeral peri-arthritis (frozen shoulder), and hyperhidrosis.

Stratified anatomy 1. skin; 2. subcutaneous tissue; 3. deltoid muscle; 4. subdeltoid bursa; 5. supraspinatus tendon.

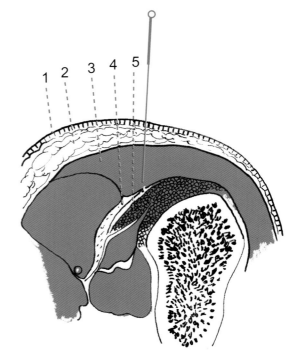

Sagittal sectional figure of LI-15 Jianyu (left)

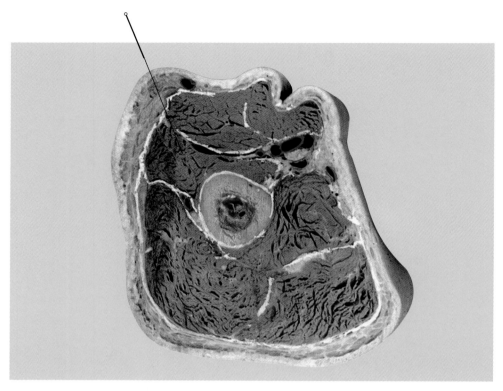

Fig. 5-1 (2) Transverse sectional figure of LU-4 Xiabai

LU-4 Xiabai

Location On the anterolateral side of the upper arm, on the radial border of the biceps brachii muscle, 5 cun proximal to LU-5 Chize and 1 cun distal to LU-3 Tianfu.

Method Insert perpendicularly 0.7 cun.

Actions Regulates Qi and Blood, alleviates pain.

Indications Epistaxis, facial paralysis, tonsillitis, and neuralgia of the forearms.

Stratified anatomy 1. skin; 2. subcutaneous tissue; 3. brachialis muscle.

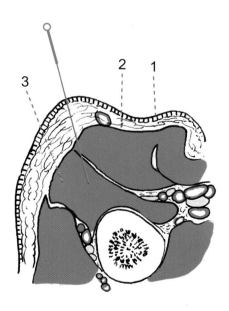

Transverse sectional figure of LU-4 Xiabai (left)

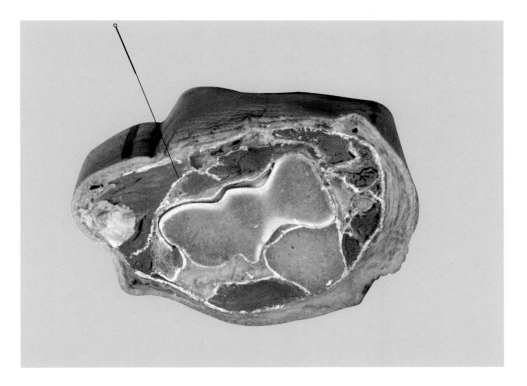

Fig. 5-1 (3) Transverse sectional figure of LU-5 Chize (left)

LU-5 Chize

Location On the cubital crease, in the depression at the radial side of the tendon of the biceps brachii.

Method Insert perpendicularly 0.7 cun.

Actions Clears Heat from the Lungs and bears counterflow Qi downward.

Indications Pneumonia, bronchitis, pleurisy, swelling and pain in the throat, swelling and pain in the elbow and arm, and erysipelas.

Stratified anatomy 1. skin; 2. subcutaneous tissue; 3. brachioradialis muscle; 4. radial nerve and anterior branch of the radial collateral artery; 5. brachialis muscle.

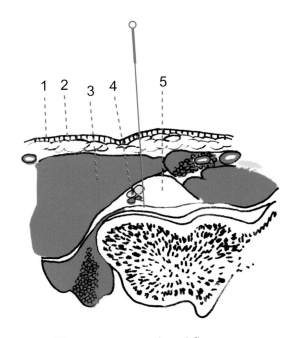

Transverse sectional figure
of LU-5 Chize (left)

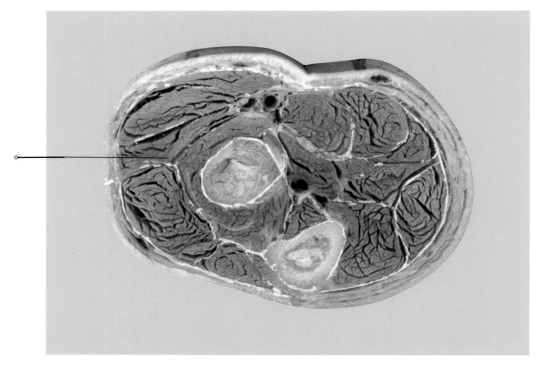

Fig. 5-1 (4) Transverse sectional figure of LI-10 Shousanli (left)

LI-10 Shousanli

Location On the radial side of the posterior surface of the forearm, on the line connecting LI-5 Yangxi and LI-11 Quchi, 2 cun distal to LI-11 Quchi.

Method Insert perpendicularly 0.8 cun.

Actions Invigorates the channels and harmonizes the Intestines.

Indications Pain in the shoulder and arm, paralysis of the upper limbs, ulcerative diseases, abdominal pain, diarrhea, and dyspepsia.

Stratified anatomy 1. skin; 2. subcutaneous tissue; 3. extensor carpi radialis longus muscle; 4. extensor carpi radialis brevis muscle; 5. extensor digitorum communis muscle; 6. supinator muscle; 7. deep branches of the radial nerve.

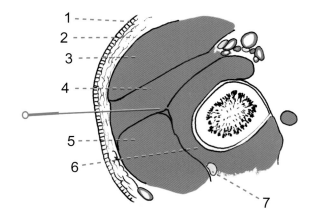

Transverse sectional figure
of LI-10 Shousanli (left)

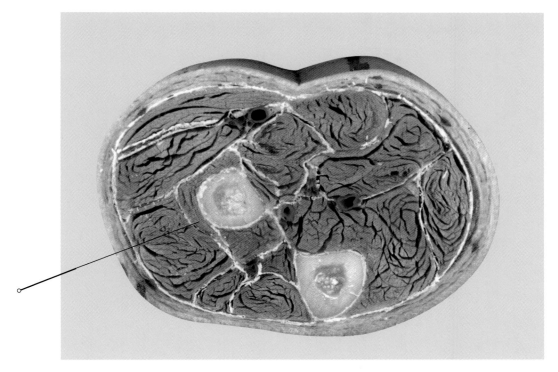

Fig. 5-1 (5) Transverse sectional figure of LI-9 Shanglian (left)

LI-9 Shanglian

Location On the radial side of the posterior surface of the forearm, on the line connecting LI-5 Yangxi and LI-11 Quchi, 3 cun distal to LI-11 Quchi.

Method Insert perpendicularly 1.3 cun.

Actions Invigorates the channels, alleviates pain, and harmonizes the Large Intestine.

Indications Hemiplegia, sprain in the forearm, numbness of the hands and feet, and abdominal pain.

Stratified anatomy 1. skin; 2. subcutaneous tissue; 3. extensor carpi radialis brevis muscle; 4. supinator muscle; 5. abductor pollicis longus muscle.

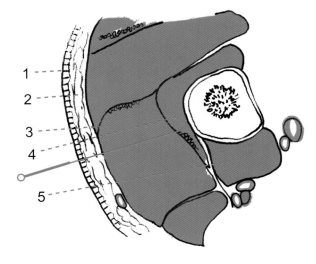

Transverse sectional figure
of LI-9 Shanglian (left)

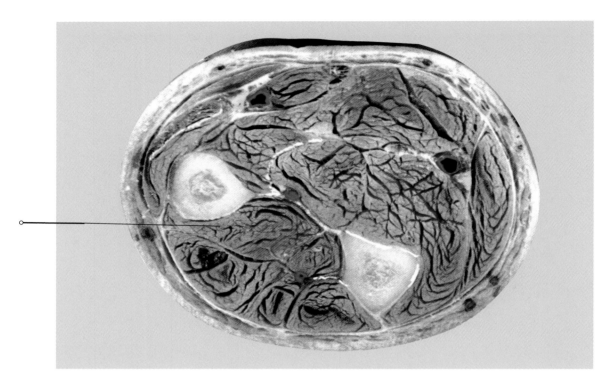

Fig. 5-1 (6) Transverse sectional figure of LI-8 Xialian (left)

LI-8 Xialian

Location On the radial side of the posterior surface of the forearm, on the line connecting LI-5 Yangxi and LI-11 Quchi, 4 cun distal to LI-11 Quchi.

Method Insert perpendicularly 0.8 cun.

Actions Clears Heat, calms the Spirit, expels Wind, and alleviates pain.

Indications Headache, pain in the eyes, dizziness, abdominal pain, mastitis, and pain in the elbow and arm.

Stratified anatomy 1. skin; 2. subcutaneous tissue. 3; brachioradialis muscle: 4. extensor carpi radialis brevis muscle; 5. supinator muscle.

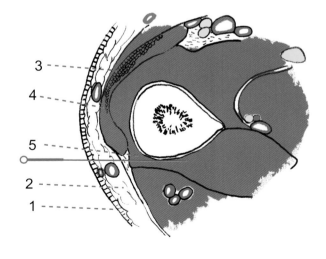

Transverse sectional figure of LI-8 Xialian (left)

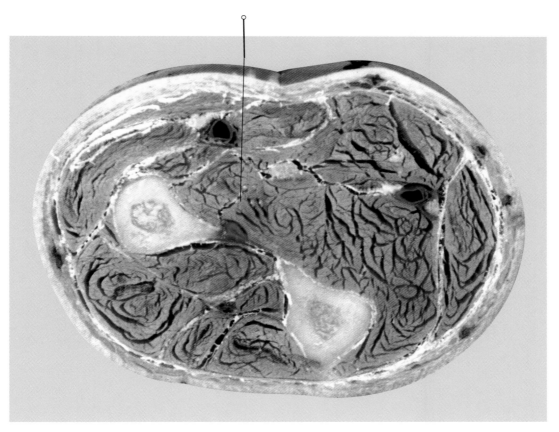

Fig. 5-1 (7) Transverse sectional figure of LU-6 Kongzui (left)

LU-6 Kongzui

Location On the anterior side of the forearm, on the line connecting LU-9 Taiyuan and LU-5 Chize, 7 cun proximal to LU-9 Taiyuan.

Method Insert perpendicularly 0.8-1 cun.

Actions Regulates and bears Lung Qi downward, clears Heat, and stops bleeding.

Indications Cough, asthma, pneumonia, and tonsillitis.

Stratified anatomy 1. skin; 2. subcutaneous tissue; 3. brachioradialis muscle; 4. flexor carpi radialis muscle; 5. flexor digitorum superficialis and pronator teres muscles; 6. flexor pollicis longus muscle.

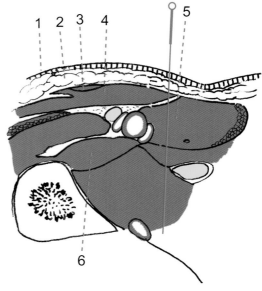

Transverse sectional figure
of LU-6 Kongzui (left)

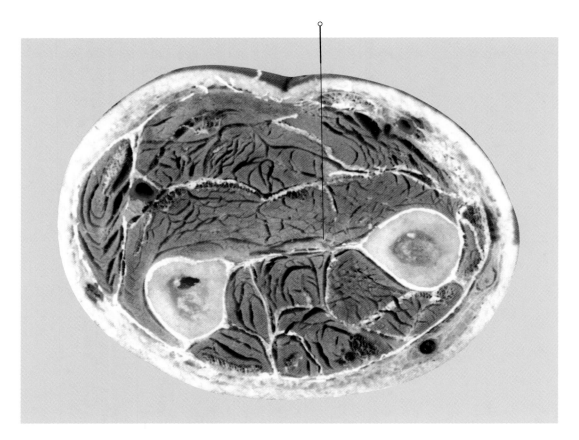

Fig. 5-1 (8) Transverse sectional figure of Bizhong (left)

Bizhong

Location On the anterior side of the forearm, between the radius and ulna, at the midpoint of the line connecting the transverse crease of the wrist and the cubital crease.

Method Insert perpendicularly 1.2 cun.

Actions Invigorates the channels, regulates Qi and calms the Spirit.

Indications Pain in the forearm, upper limb paralysis or spasm, anxiety disorder, and pain in the chest and hypochondrium.

Stratified anatomy 1. skin; 2. subcutaneous tissue; 3. flexor carpi radialis muscle; 4. flexor digitorum superficialis muscle; 5. median nerve and artery; 6. flexor digitorum profundus muscle.

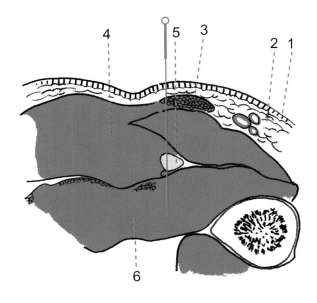

Transverse sectional figure of Bizhong (left)

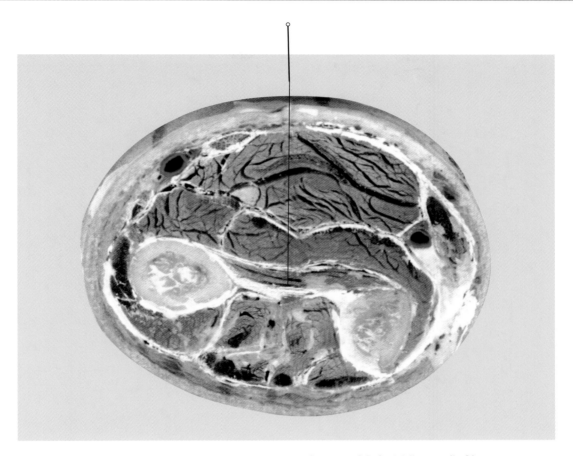

Fig. 5-1 (9) Transverse sectional figure of PC-4 Ximen (left)

PC-4 Ximen

Location On the anterior aspect of the forearm, on the line connecting PC-7 Daling and PC-3 Quze, 5 cun proximal to PC-7 Daling.

Method Insert perpendicularly 0.8-1 cun.

Actions Calms the Spirit, regulates Qi and Blood.

Indications Rheumatic heart disease, myocarditis, angina pectoris, palpitations, mastitis, pleurisy, phrenospasm, and anxiety disorder.

Stratified anatomy 1. skin. 2. subcutaneous tissue; 3. flexor carpi radialis muscle; 4. flexor digitorum superficialis muscle; 5. median nerve and artery; 6. flexor digitorum profundus muscle; 7. anterior aspect of the interosseous membrane of the forearm.

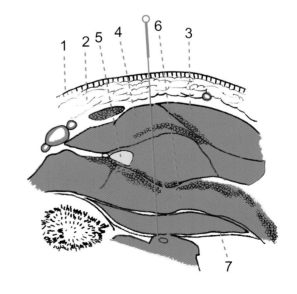

Transverse sectional figure of PC-4 Ximen (left)

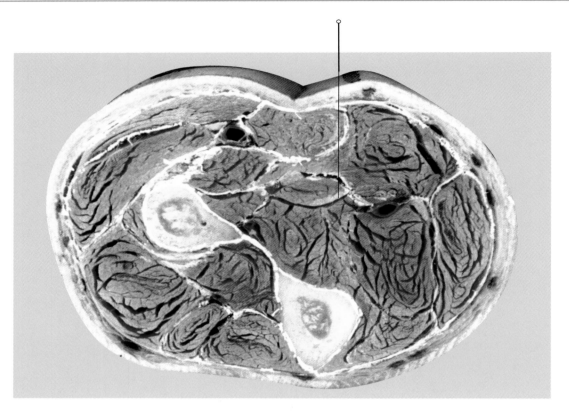

Fig. 5-1 (10) Transverse sectional figure of EX-UE-2 Erbai (medial, left)

EX-UE-2 Erbai

Location On the anterior aspect of the forearm, 4 cun proximal to PC-7 Daling, on each side of the tendon of the flexor carpi radialis muscle, two points in total.

Method Insert perpendicularly 1 cun at the medial point and 0.5 cun at the lateral point.

Actions Regulates Qi, alleviates pain, treats hemorrhoids, and bears Qi upward.

Indications Hemorrhoids, proctoptosis, pain in the forearm, and pain in the chest and hypochondrium.

Stratified anatomy The medial acupuncture point: 1. skin; 2. subcutaneous tissue; 3. the space between the palmaris longus and flexor carpi radialis muscles; 4. flexor digitorum superficialis muscle; 5. median nerve and artery; 6. flexor pollicis longus muscle; 7. anterior aspect of the interosseous membrane of the forearm.

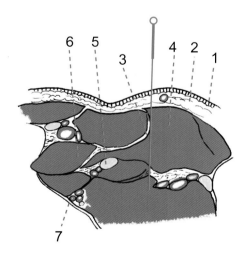

Transverse sectional figure of EX-UE-2 Erbai (medial, left)

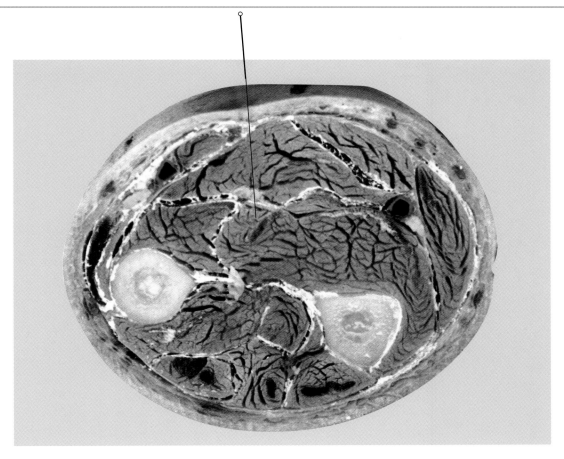

Fig. 5-1 (11) Transverse sectional figure of PC-5 Jianshi (left)

PC-5 Jianshi

Location On the anterior aspect of the forearm, 3 cun proximal to the midpoint of the transverse carpal crease, between the tendons of the flexor carpi radialis and palmaris longus muscles.

Method Insert perpendicularly 0.8 cun.

Actions Calms the Spirit, eliminates Phlegm and harmonizes the Stomach.

Indications Rheumatic heart disease, stomachache, malaria, epilepsy, anxiety disorder, and schizophrenia.

Stratified anatomy 1. skin; 2. subcutaneous tissue; 3. the tendons of (a) the palmaris longus muscle and (b) the flexor carpi radialis muscle; 4. flexor digitorum superficialis muscle; 5. flexor digitorum profundus muscle; 6. pronator quadratus muscle; 7. anterior aspect of the interosseous membrane of the forearm.

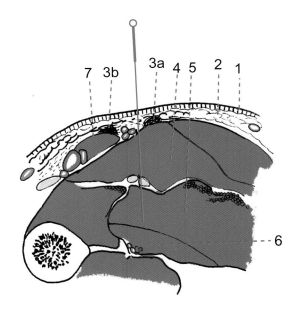

Transverse sectional figure
of PC-5 Jianshi (left)

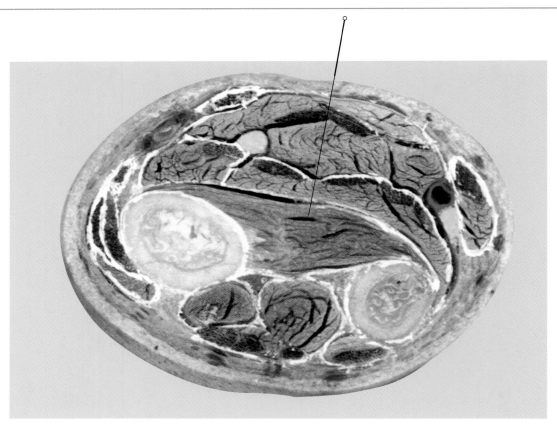

Fig. 5-1 (12) Transverse sectional figure of PC-6 Neiguan (left)

PC-6 Neiguan

Location On the anterior aspect of the forearm, 2 cun superior to the transverse carpal crease, between the tendons of the flexor carpi radialis and palmaris longus muscles.

Method Insert perpendicularly 1 cun.

Actions Regulates chest and Stomach Qi and calms the Spirit.

Indications Rheumatic heart disease, shock, angina pectoris, palpitations, vomiting, chest pain, stomachache, abdominal pain, phrenospasm, migraine, hyperthyroidism, epilepsy, anxiety disorder, asthma, swelling and pain in the throat, and postoperative pain.

Stratified anatomy 1. skin; 2. subcutaneous tissue; 3. tendons of (a) the palmaris longus muscle and (b) the flexor carpi radialis muscle; 4. flexor digitorum superficialis muscle; 5. median nerve and artery; 6. flexor digitorum profundus muscle; 7. pronator quadratus muscle.

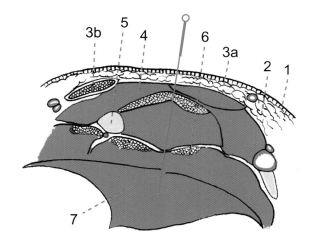

Transverse sectional figure
of PC-6 Neiguan (left)

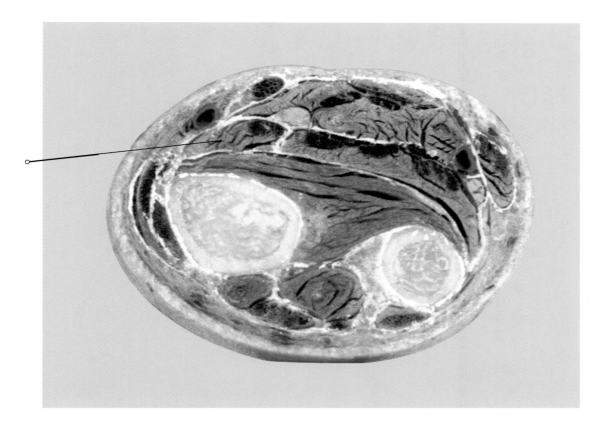

Fig. 5-1 (13) Transverse sectional figure of LU-7 Lieque (left)

LU-7 Lieque

Location Proximal to the styloid process of the radius, 1.5 cun above the transverse carpal crease, between the tendons of the brachioradialis and abductor pollicis longus muscles.

Method Insert transversely 0.3 cun.

Actions Opens and regulates the Conception vessel and the Lungs, dispels Wind and alleviates pain.

Indications Urticaria, facial paralysis, stiffness and pain in the neck, and soft tissue diseases of the carpal periarticulation.

Stratified anatomy 1. skin; 2. subcutaneous tissue; 3. abductor pollicis longus tendon; 4. brachioradialis tendon; 5. pronator quadratus muscle.

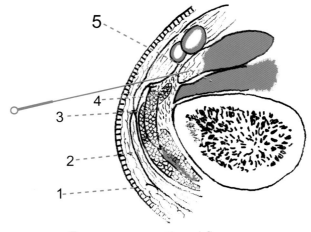

Transverse sectional figure of LU-7 Lieque (left)

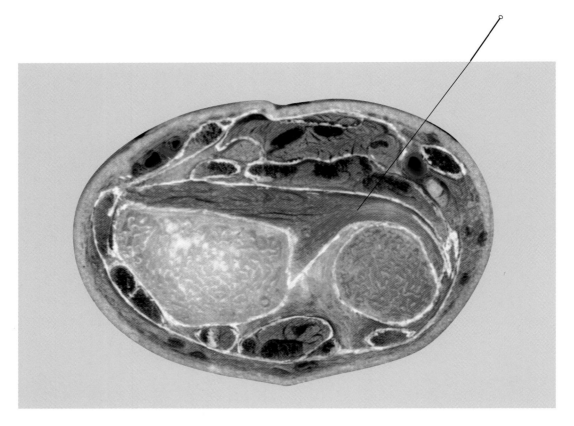

Fig. 5-1 (14) Transverse sectional figure of HT-5 Tongli (left)

HT-5 Tongli

Location On the anterior aspect of the forearm, 1 cun proximal to the transverse carpal crease (HT-7 Shenmen), on the radial side of the tendon of the flexor carpi ulnaris muscle.

Method Insert perpendicularly 0.8 cun.

Actions Calms the Spirit, regulates Heart Qi, and benefits the tongue.

Indications Palpitations, angina pectoris, bradycardia, neurasthenia, functional aphasia, schizophrenia, cough, and asthma.

Stratified anatomy 1. skin; 2. subcutaneous tissue; 3. radial side of the flexor carpi ulnaris muscle; 4. ulnar side of the flexor digitorum profundus muscle; 5. posterior space of the flexor muscles of the forearm; 6. pronator quadratus muscle; 7. posterior interosseous artery, vein and nerve.

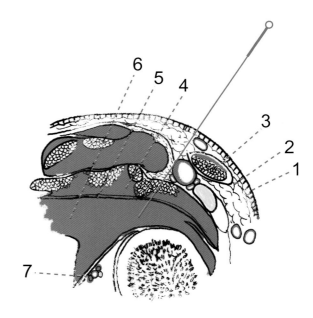

Transverse sectional figure
of HT-5 Tongli (left)

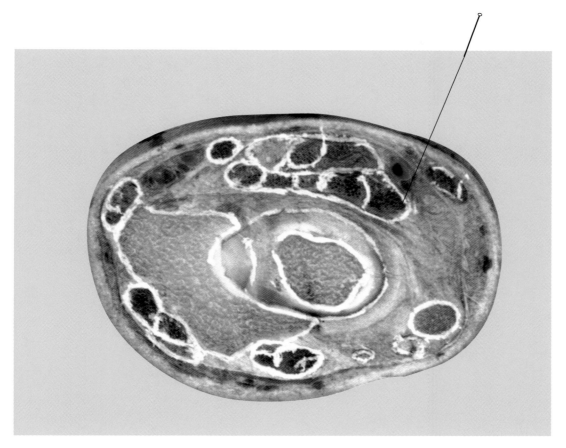

Fig. 5-1 (15) Transverse sectional figure of HT-6 Yinxi (left)

HT-6 Yinxi

Location On the anterior aspect of the forearm, 0.5 cun above the transverse carpal crease (HT-7 Shenmen), on the radial side of the tendon of the flexor carpi ulnaris muscle.

Method Insert perpendicularly 0.4 cun.

Actions Regulates Heart Qi and Blood, clears Deficiency-Fire.

Indications Neurasthenia, night sweating, palpitations, and pulmonary tuberculosis.

Stratified anatomy 1. skin; 2. subcutaneous tissue; 3. radial side of the tendon of the flexor carpi ulnaris muscle; 4. ulnar nerve.

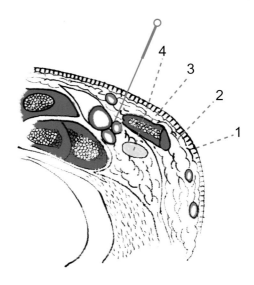

Transverse sectional figure
of HT-6 Yinxi (left)

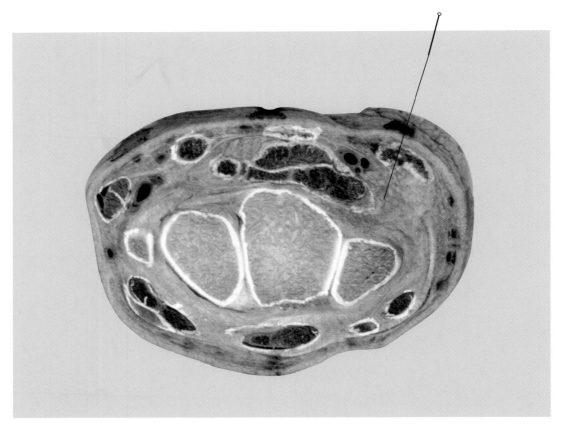

Fig. 5-1 (16) Transverse sectional figure of HT-7 Shenmen (left)

HT-7 Shenmen

Location On the anterior side, at the ulnar end of the transverse carpal crease, on the radial side of the tendon of the flexor carpi ulnaris muscle, in the depression at the proximal border of the pisiform bone.

Method Insert perpendicularly 0.5 cun.

Actions Calms the Spirit, regulates and supplements the Heart, and dredges the channels.

Indications Neurasthenia, palpitations, amnesia, insomnia, dreaminess, heart disease, angina pectoris, anxiety disorder, and paralysis of the muscles of the tongue.

Stratified anatomy 1. skin; 2. subcutaneous tissue; 3. ulnar side: tendon of the flexor carpi ulnaris muscle; 4. radial side: ulnar nerve, artery and vein.

Cautions The ulnar artery and ulnar nerve lie adjacent to this point.

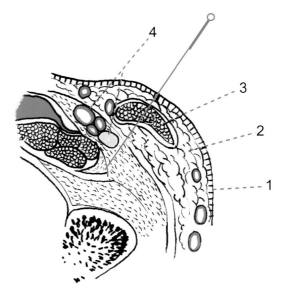

Transverse sectional figure
of HT-7 Shenmen (left)

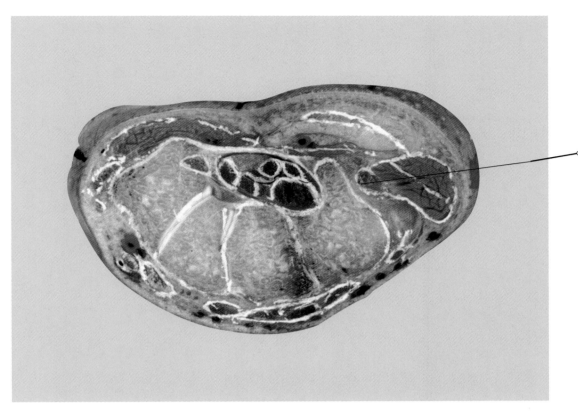

Fig. 5-1 (17) Transverse sectional figure of SI-4 Wangu (left)

SI-4 Wangu

Location On the ulnar side of the wrist, in the depression between the 5th metacarpal bone and the triquetral bone.

Method Insert perpendicularly 0.8 cun.

Actions Clears Heat and Damp-Heat, invigorates the channels and alleviates pain.

Indications Arthritis of the wrist, elbow and fingers, headache, and tinnitus.

Stratified anatomy 1. skin; 2. subcutaneous tissue; 3. abductor digiti minimi muscle; 4. pisometacarpal ligament; 5. tendon of the extensor carpi ulnaris muscle and the base of the fifth metacarpal.

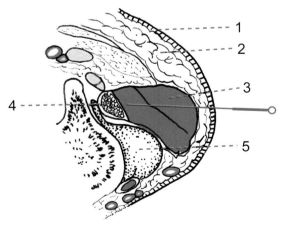

Transverse sectional figure of SI-4 Wangu (left)

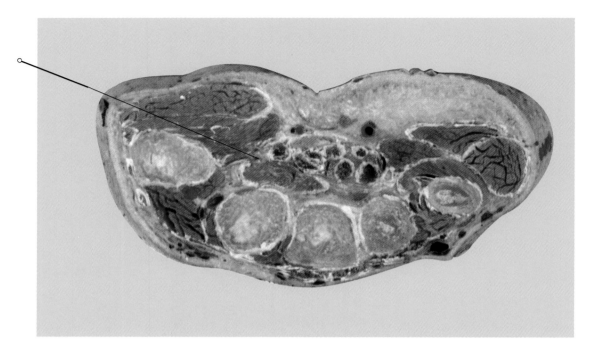

Fig. 5-1 (18) Transverse sectional figure of LU-10 Yuji (left)

LU-10 Yuji

Location At the junction of the radial palmar and dorsal aspects, at the midpoint of the first metacarpal bone.

Method Insert perpendicularly 1 cun toward the palm.

Actions Clears Lung-Heat, benefits the throat, and bears counterflow Qi downward.

Indications Sore throat, tonsillitis, asthma, hemoptysis, and infantile malnutrition.

Stratified anatomy 1. skin; 2. subcutaneous tissue; 3. abductor pollicis brevis muscle; 4. opponens pollicis muscle; 5. flexor pollicis brevis muscle.

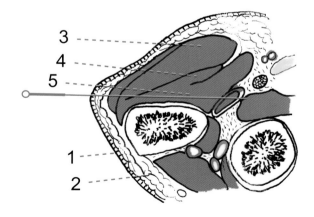

Transverse sectional figure
of LU-10 Yuji (left)

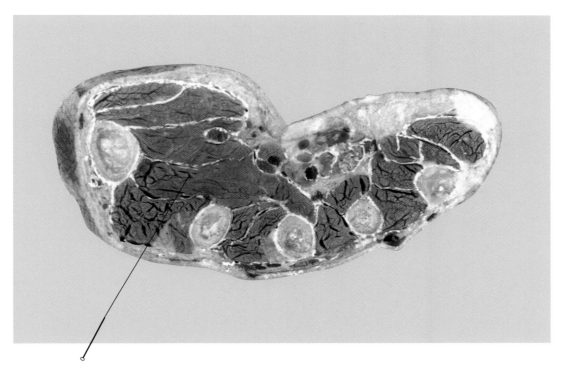

Fig. 5-1 (19) Transverse sectional figure of LI-4 Hegu (left)

LI-4 Hegu

Location On the dorsum of the hand, between the first and second metacarpal bones, approximately at the midpoint of the second metacarpal bone.

Method Insert perpendicularly 0.8 cun.

Actions Disperses Wind, releases the exterior, invigorates the channels, and alleviates pain.

Indications Common cold, diseases of the ear, eye, nose and throat, facial paralysis, hemiplegia, neurasthenia, and various painful conditions.

Stratified anatomy 1. skin; 2. subcutaneous tissue; 3. first dorsal interosseous muscle; 4. adductor pollicis muscle.

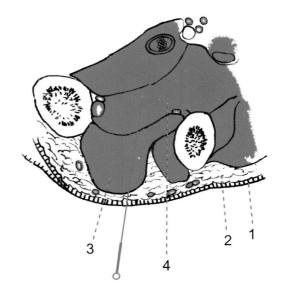

Transverse sectional figure
of LI-4 Hegu (left)

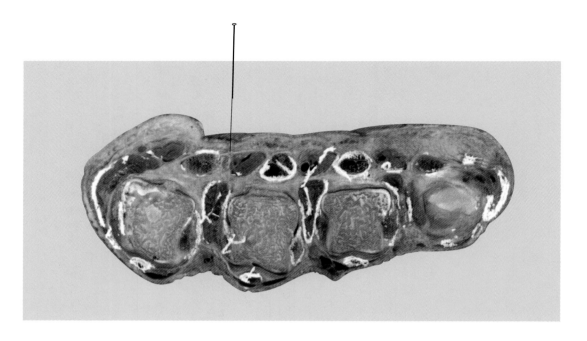

Fig. 5-1 (20) Transverse sectional figure of PC-8 Laogong (left)

PC-8 Laogong

Location Between the second and third metacarpal bones, adjacent to the third metacarpal bone, proximal to the transverse palmar crease.

Method Insert perpendicularly 0.4 cun.

Actions Clears Heat from Heart, Pericardium and Blood, and calms the Spirit.

Indications Apoplexy, coma, sunstroke, angina pectoris, stomatitis, infantile convulsions, anxiety disorder, psychosis, hyperhidrosis of the palm, and numbness of the fingers.

Stratified anatomy 1. skin; 2. subcutaneous tissue; 3. palmar aponeurosis; 4. between the tendons of the flexor superficialis digitorum and flexor profundus muscles on the radial side; 5. radial side of the second lumbrical muscle, the common palmar digital artery and the proper palmar digital nerve; 6. first palmar interosseous muscle and the second dorsal interosseous muscle.

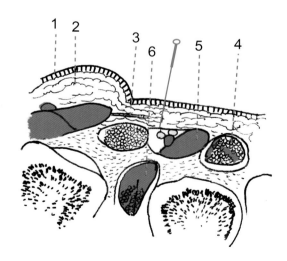

Transverse sectional figure
of PC-8 Laogong (left)

ACUPUNCTURE POINTS ON THE LEG AND FOOT

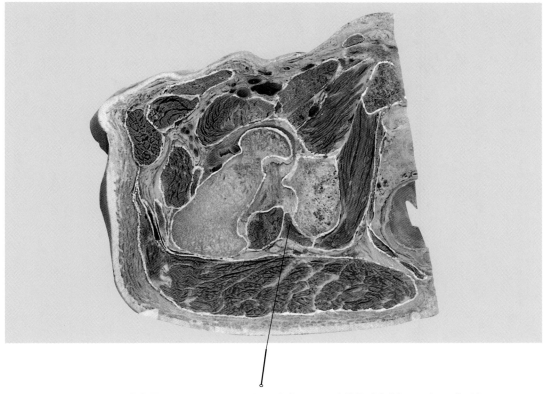

Fig. 5-2 (1) Transverse sectional figure of GB-30 Huantiao (left)

GB-30 Huantiao

Location At the junction of the medial 2/3 and lateral 1/3 of the line connecting the prominence of the greater trochanter and the sacral hiatus.

Method Insert perpendicularly 2-2.5 cun.

Actions Benefits the lower back and legs, invigorates the channels, and alleviates pain.

Indications Sciatica, palsy or paralysis of the lower limbs, and diseases of the hip joint and periarticular soft tissue.

Stratified anatomy 1. skin; 2. subcutaneous tissue; 3. gluteus maximus muscle; 4. sciatic nerve; 5. quadratus femoris muscle.

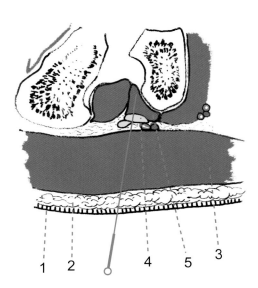

Transverse sectional figure
of GB-30 Huantiao (left)

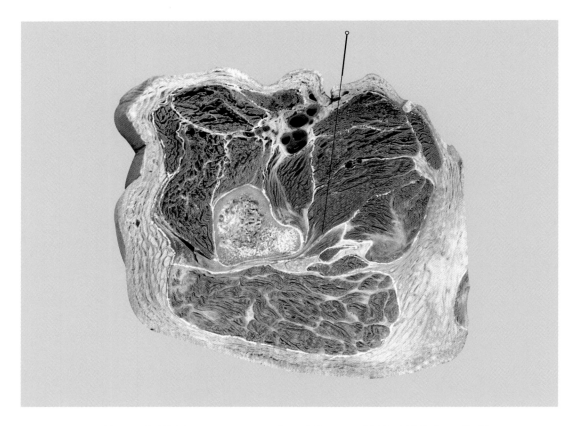

Fig. 5-2 (2) Transverse sectional figure of LR-11 Yinlian (left)

LR-11 Yinlian

Location 2 cun inferior and 2 cun lateral to CV-2 Qugu.

Method Insert perpendicularly 1-1.5 cun.

Actions Benefits the Uterus.

Indications Irregular menstruation, pain in the lower back and legs, and pain due to hernia.

Stratified anatomy 1. skin; 2. subcutaneous tissue; 3. adductor longus muscle; 4. adductor brevis muscle; 5. adductor minimus muscle.

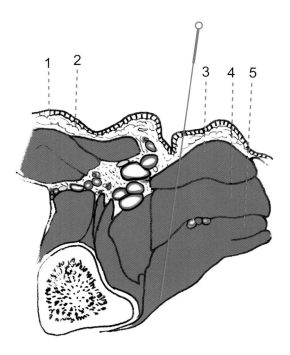

Transverse sectional figure of LR-11 Yinlian (left)

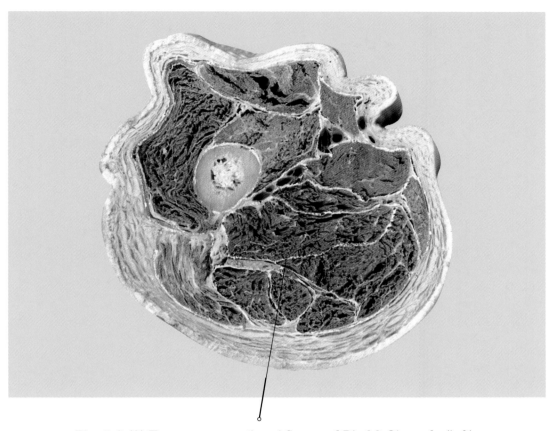

Fig. 5-2 (3) Transverse sectional figure of BL-36 Chengfu (left)

BL-36 Chengfu

Location On the inferior border of the gluteus maximus muscle on the midline of the posterior thigh.

Method Insert perpendicularly 1.5-2 cun.

Actions Regulates the Lower Burner and alleviates pain.

Indications Lumbago, sciatica, hemorrhoids, retention of urine, and constipation.

Stratified anatomy 1. skin; 2. subcutaneous tissue; 3. gluteus maximus muscle; 4. trunk of the posterior cutaneous nerve of the thigh; 5. long head of the biceps femoris muscle and the semitendinosus muscle; 6. sciatic nerve and its accompanying artery.

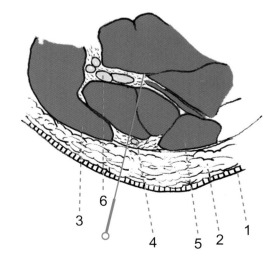

Transverse sectional figure
of BL-36 Chengfu (left)

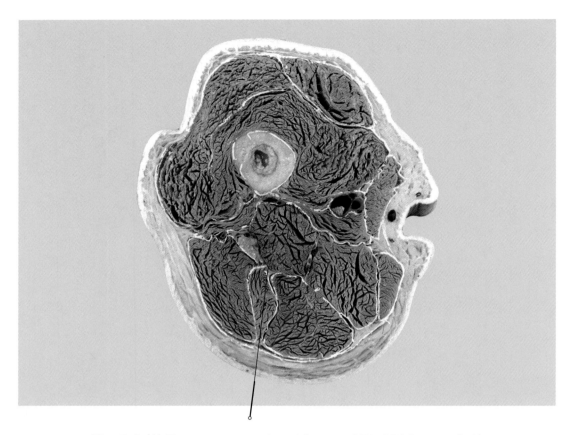

Fig. 5-2 (4) Transverse sectional figure of BL-37 Yinmen (left)

BL-37 Yinmen

Location Inferior to the midpoint of the gluteal crease, 6 cun below BL-36 Chengfu.

Method Insert perpendicularly 1.5-2 cun.

Actions Invigorates the channels, alleviates pain, and benefits the lower back.

Indications Lumbago, sciatica, paraparesis, and occipital headache.

Stratified anatomy 1. skin; 2. subcutaneous tissue; 3. long head of the biceps femoris muscle and the semitendinosus muscle; 4. sciatic nerve and its accompanying artery.

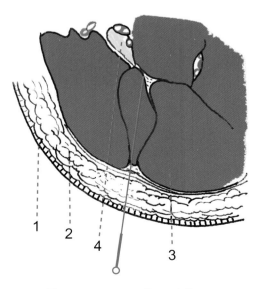

Transverse sectional figure
of BL-37 Yinmen (left)

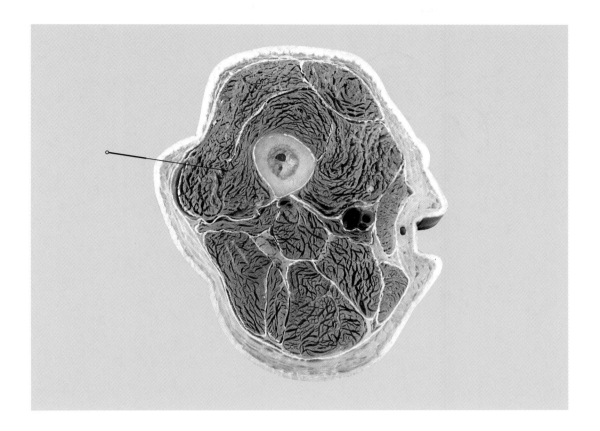

Fig. 5-2 (5) Transverse sectional figure of GB-31 Fengshi (left)

GB-31 Fengshi

Location On the line connecting the prominence of the greater trochanter and the head of the fibula, 12 cun inferior to the prominence of the greater trochanter, 7 cun superior to the popliteal crease.

Method Insert perpendicularly 1-2 cun.

Actions Invigorates the channels, alleviates pain, and expels Wind.

Indications Paralysis of the lower limbs, lumbago, and neuritis of the lateral cutaneous nerve of the thigh.

Stratified anatomy 1. skin; 2. subcutaneous tissue; 3. iliotibial tract; 4. vastus lateralis muscle; 5. vastus intermedius muscle.

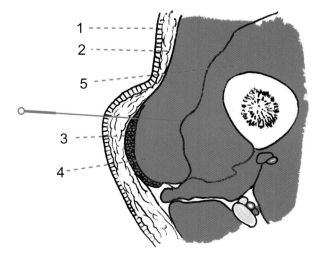

Transverse sectional figure
of GB-31 Fengshi (left)

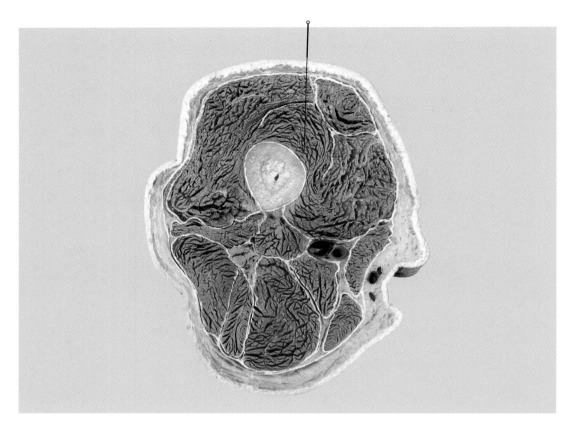

Fig. 5-2 (6) Transverse sectional figure of ST-32 Futu (left)

ST-32 Futu

Location With the knee extended, on the line connecting the anterior superior iliac spine and ST-35 Dubi, 6 cun superior to the superior border of the patella.

Method Insert perpendicularly 1-2 cun.

Actions Invigorates the channels, alleviates pain, and expels Wind-Damp.

Indications Paralysis and palsy of the lower limbs, inflammation of the knee, and urticaria.

Stratified anatomy 1. skin; 2. subcutaneous tissue; 3. rectus femoris muscle; 4. descending branches of the lateral circumflex artery and vein and the muscular branches of the femoral nerve; 5. vastus intermedius muscle.

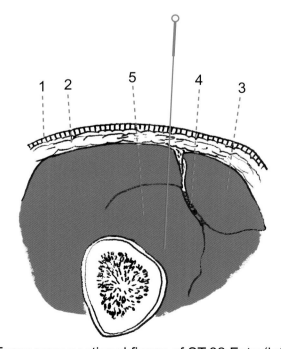

Transverse sectional figure of ST-32 Futu (left)

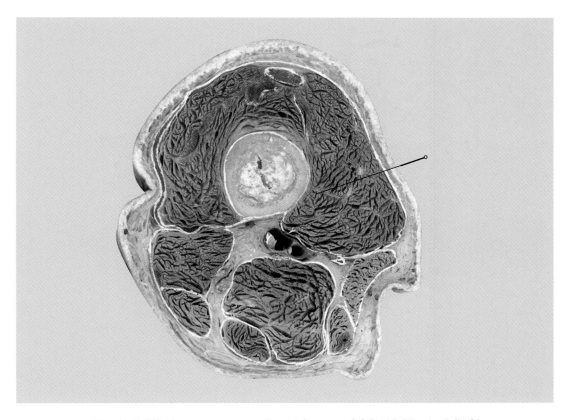

Fig. 5-2 (7) Transverse sectional figure of SP-10 Xuehai (left)

SP-10 Xuehai

Location On the anterior inferior part of the medial aspect of the thigh, on the prominence of the vastus medialis muscle, 2 cun superior to the upper border of the patella.

Method Insert perpendicularly 1 cun.

Actions Invigorates Qi and Blood and clears Heat.

Indications Irregular menstruation, dysfunctional uterine bleeding, urticaria, pruritus, neurodermatitis, and anemia.

Stratified anatomy 1. skin; 2. subcutaneous tissue; 3. vastus medialis muscle.

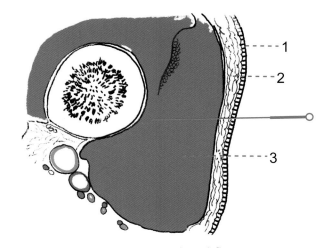

Transverse sectional figure
of SP-10 Xuehai (left)

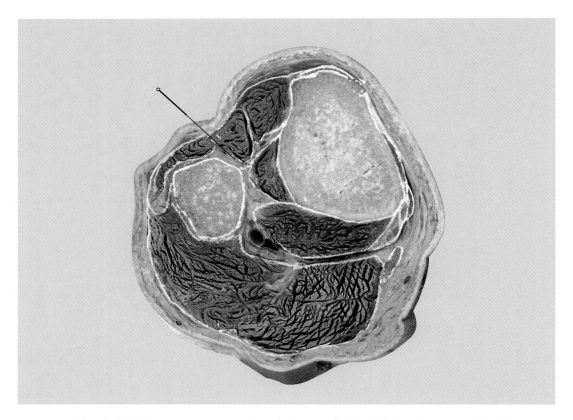

Fig. 5-2 (8) Transverse sectional figure of GB-34 Yanglingquan (left)

GB-34 Yanglingquan

Location In the depression anterior and inferior to the head of the fibula, at the tibio-fibular articulation.

Method Insert perpendicularly 1-1.5 cun.

Actions Benefits the Liver and Gallbladder, clears Damp-Heat and strengthens the sinews and bones.

Indications Hepatitis, cholecystitis, biliary ascariasis, hypertension, intercostal neuralgia, scapulohumeral periarthritis (frozen shoulder), pain in the knee joint, paralysis of the lower limbs, numbness in the lower limbs, and habitual constipation.

Stratified anatomy 1. skin; 2. subcutaneous tissue; 3. peroneus longus muscle; 4. extensor digitorum longus muscle.

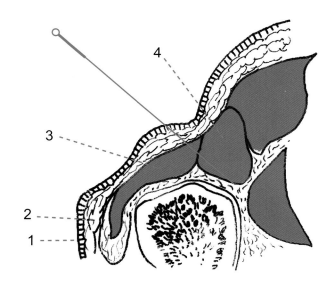

Transverse sectional figure
of GB-34 Yanglingquan (left)

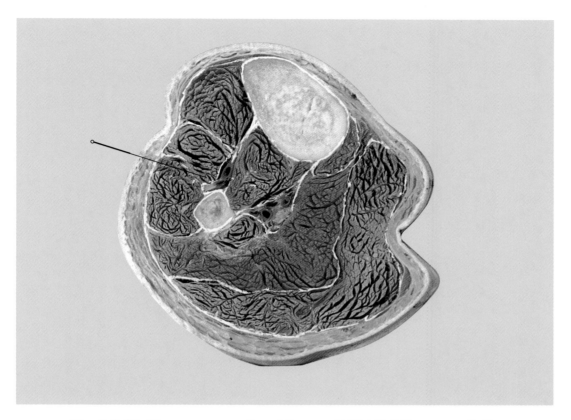

Fig. 5-2 (9) Transverse sectional figure of EX-LE-6 Dannang (left)

EX-LE-6 Dannang

Location 2 cun inferior to Yanglingquan (GB-34).

Method Insert perpendicularly 1 cun.

Actions Clears Heat and drains Dampness.

Indications Acute and chronic cholecystitis, cholelithiasis, biliary ascariasis, gallbladder colic, and pain in the hypochondrium.

Stratified anatomy 1. skin; 2. subcutaneous tissue; 3. peroneus longus muscle; 4. anterior to the superficial peroneal nerve; 5. in the deep layer, the deep peroneal nerve and the anterior tibial artery and vein.

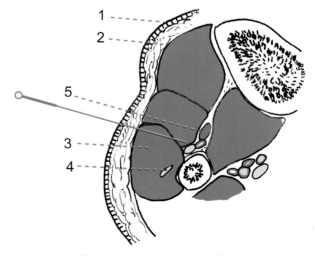

Transverse sectional figure of
EX-LE-6 Dannang (left)

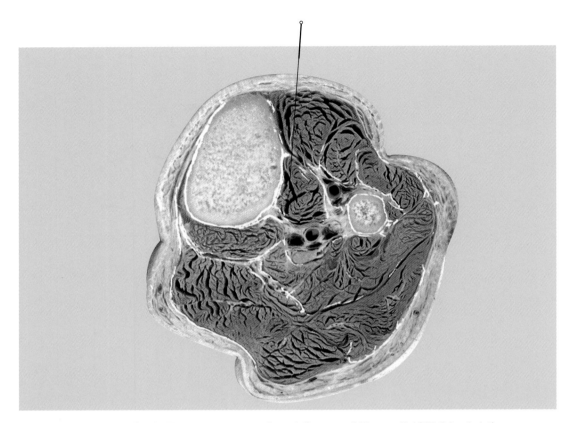

Fig. 5-2 (10) Transverse sectional figure of Zusanli (ST 36, right)

ST-36 Zusanli

Location 3 cun inferior to ST-35 Dubi, in the depression one finger-breadth lateral to the anterior crest of the tibia.

Method Insert perpendicularly 1 cun.

Actions Supplements Qi, Blood and Yin, benefits the Spleen and Stomach, invigorates the channels, and alleviates pain.

Indications Acute and chronic gastritis, ulcers, acute and chronic enteritis, acute and chronic pancreatitis, infantile dyspepsia, hemiplegia, shock, debility, anemia, hypertension, allergic diseases, jaundice, epilepsy, and neurasthenia.

Stratified anatomy 1. skin; 2. subcutaneous tissue; 3. tibialis anterior muscle; 4. interosseous membrane of the leg; 5. tibialis posterior muscle.

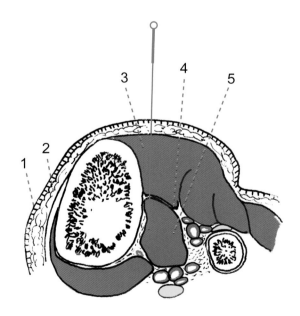

Transverse sectional figure of Zusanli (ST 36, right)

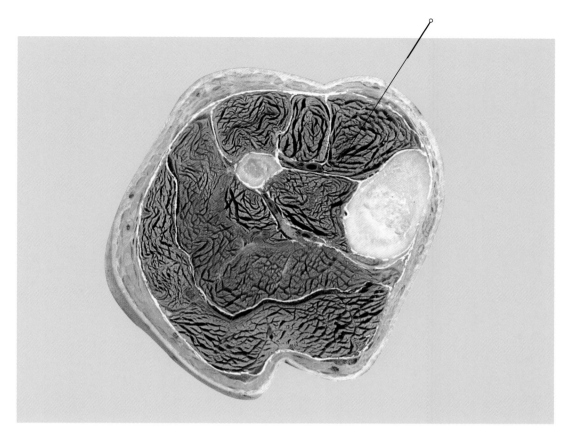

Fig. 5-2 (11) Transverse sectional figure of EX-LE-7 Lanwei (left)

EX-LE-7 Lanwei

Location 2 cun inferior to ST-36 Zusanli, 5 cun below ST-35 Dubi.

Method Insert perpendicularly 1-1.5 cun.

Actions Moves Qi and invigorates the Blood, clears Heat and Fire Toxins from the Large Intestine.

Indications Abdominal pain, abdominal distension, diarrhea, appendicitis, enteritis, bacillary dysentery, gastritis, hemiplegia, and beriberi.

Stratified anatomy 1. skin; 2. subcutaneous tissue; 3. tibialis anterior muscle; 4. anterior tibial artery and vein and deep peroneal nerve lateral to the needle; 5. interosseous membrane of the leg; 6. tibialis posterior muscle.

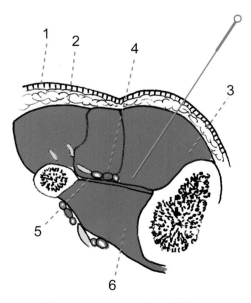

Transverse sectional figure
of EX-LE-7 Lanwei (left)

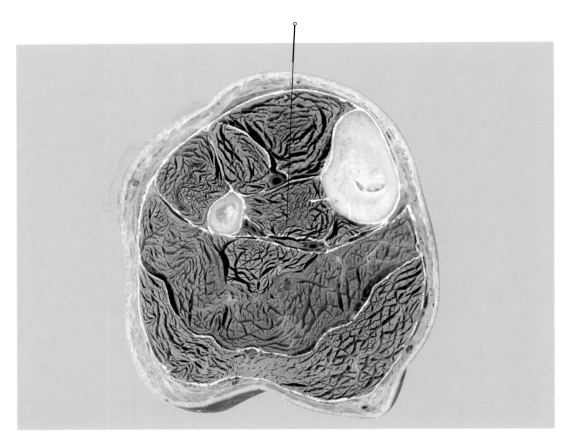

Fig. 5-2 (12) Transverse sectional figure of ST-37 Shangjuxu (left)

ST-37 Shangjuxu
Location 3 cun inferior to ST-36 Zusanli, on the tibialis anterior muscle between the tibia and fibula.

Method Insert perpendicularly 1-1.5 cun.

Actions Clears Damp-Heat, regulates the Intestines, Spleen and Stomach, invigorates the channels, and alleviates pain.

Indications Acute appendicitis, pain in the stomach and epigastrium, dyspepsia, and flaccidity, atrophy disorders and pain of the lower limbs.

Stratified anatomy 1. skin; 2. subcutaneous tissue; 3. tibialis anterior muscle; 4. anterior tibial artery and vein and the deep peroneal nerve lateral to the needle; 5. interosseous membrane of the leg; 6. tibialis posterior muscle.

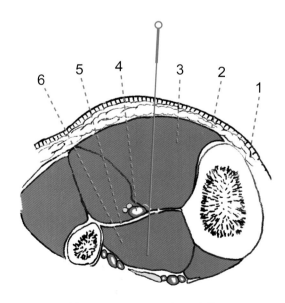

Transverse sectional figure
of ST-37 Shangjuxu (left)

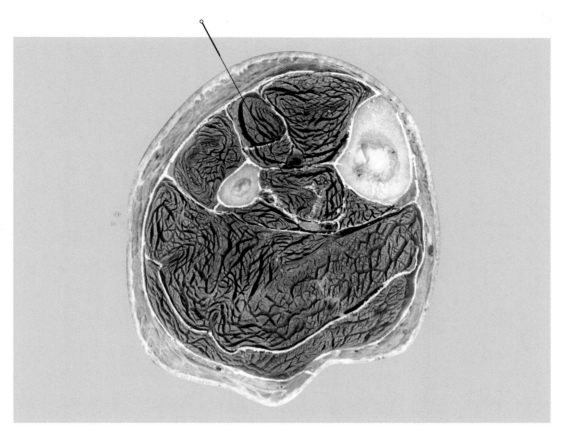

Fig. 5-2 (13) Transverse sectional figure of ST-40 Fenglong (left)

ST-40 Fenglong

Location 8 cun superior to the lateral malleolus, 1 cun lateral to ST-38 Tiaokou.

Method Insert perpendicularly 1-1.2 cun.

Actions Transforms Phlegm-Damp and calms the Spirit.

Indications Nephritis, cystitis, orchitis, pelvic infection, epilepsy, schizophrenia, and calf muscle cramp (systremma).

Stratified anatomy 1. skin; 2. subcutaneous tissue; 3. extensor digitorum longus muscle; 4. extensor hallucis longus muscle; 5. interosseous membrane of the leg; 6. tibialis posterior muscle.

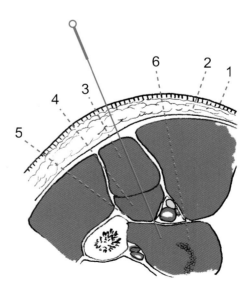

Transverse sectional figure of ST-40 Fenglong (left)

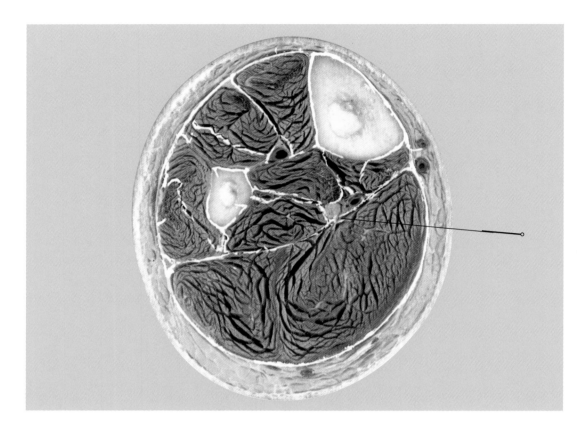

Fig. 5-2 (14) Transverse sectional figure of KI-9 Zhubin (left)

KI-9 Zhubin

Location On the medial aspect of the lower leg, 5 cun superior to KI-3 Taixi, at the junction of the middle and posterior third of the line connecting KI-3 Taixi and KI-10 Yingu.

Method Insert perpendicularly 1 cun.

Actions Regulates Qi, alleviates pain, transforms Phlegm, and calms the Spirit.

Indications Cough, profuse expectoration, headache, vertigo, beriberi, edema in the lower limb, amenorrhea, and metrorrhagia.

Stratified anatomy 1. skin; 2. subcutaneous tissue; 3. triceps surae muscle; 4. anterior medial aspect of the tendon of the plantaris muscle; 5. tibial nerve.

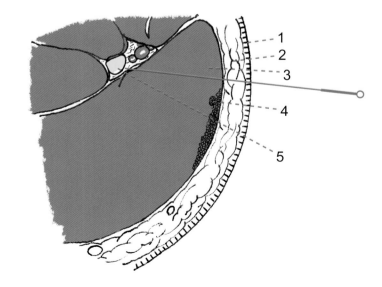

Transverse sectional figure of KI-9 Zhubin (left)

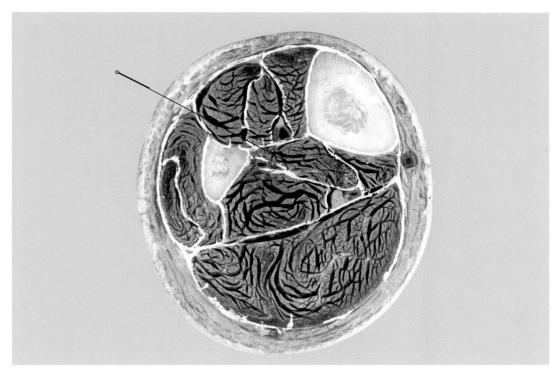

Fig. 5-2 (15) Transverse sectional figure of GB-37 Guangming (left)

GB-37 Guangming

Location On the lower part of the lateral aspect of the leg, 5 cun superior to the lateral malleolus, at the anterior border of the fibula, between the extensor digitorum longus and peroneus brevis muscles.

Method Insert perpendicularly 1 cun.

Actions Dispels Wind-Damp, alleviates pain and benefits the eyes.

Indications Night blindness, optic atrophy, cataract, migraine, and pain in the lateral aspect of the leg.

Stratified anatomy 1. skin; 2. subcutaneous tissue; 3. peroneus brevis muscle; 4. anterior intermuscular septum; 5. extensor digitorum longus muscle; 6. extensor hallucis longus muscle; 7. the anterior tibial artery and vein and the deep peroneal nerve; 8. interosseous membrane of the leg; 9. tibialis posterior muscle.

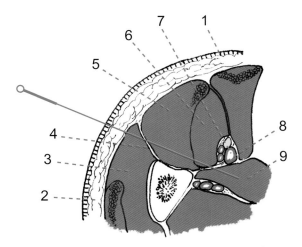

Transverse sectional figure of
GB-37 Guangming (left)

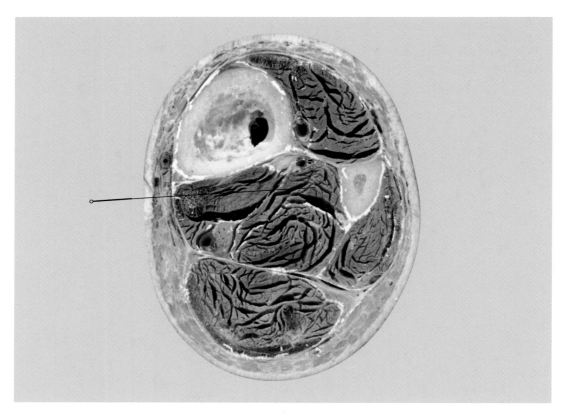

Fig. 5-2 (16) Transverse sectional figure of SP-6 Sanyinjiao (right)

SP-6 Sanyinjiao

Location On the lower part of the anterior medial aspect of the leg, 3 cun superior to the tip of the medial malleolus, in the depression posterior to the medial border of the tibia.

Method Insert perpendicularly 1-1.2 cun.

Actions Fortifies the Spleen, transforms Damp- ness, allows constrained Liver Qi to flow freely, and benefits the Kidneys.

Indications Nephritis, orchitis, dysfunctional uterine bleeding, urinary tract infection, leukor- rhea, and lumbago.

Stratified anatomy 1. skin; 2. subcutaneous tissue; 3. flexor digitorum longus muscle; 4. tibialis posterior muscle; 5. flexor hallucis longus muscle; 6. posterior tibial artery and vein; 7. anterior tibial artery and vein.

Caution Contraindicated during pregnancy.

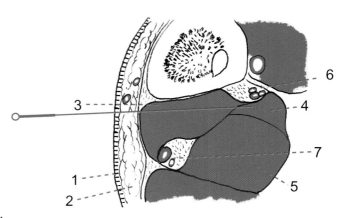

Transverse sectional figure
of SP-6 Sanyinjiao (right)

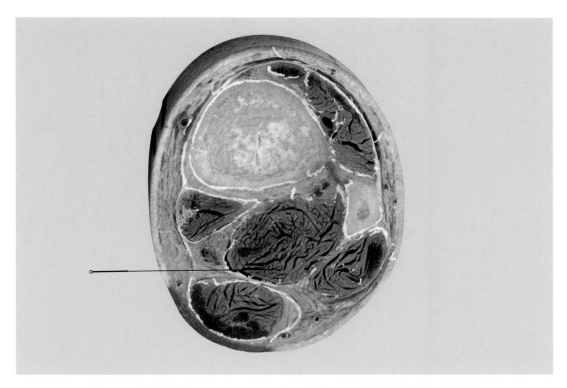

Fig. 5-2 (17) Transverse sectional figure of KI-7 Fuliu (right)

KI-7 Fuliu

Location On the lower part of the medial aspect of the leg, 2 cun superior to KI-3 Taixi, anterior to the Achilles tendon.

Method Insert perpendicularly 0.5-1 cun.

Actions Benefits the Kidneys, regulates the water passages, drains Dampness, and clears Damp-Heat.

Indications Diseases of the genito-urinary system, abdominal distension, abdominal pain, diarrhea, hemiplegia, neurasthenia, neurodermatitis, eczema, and urticaria.

Stratified anatomy 1. skin; 2. subcutaneous tissue; 3. the tendon of the plantaris muscle and the Achilles tendon; 4. the tibial nerve and the posterior tibial artery and vein; 5. flexor hallucis longus muscle.

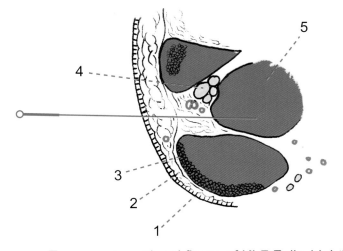

Transverse sectional figure of KI-7 Fuliu (right)

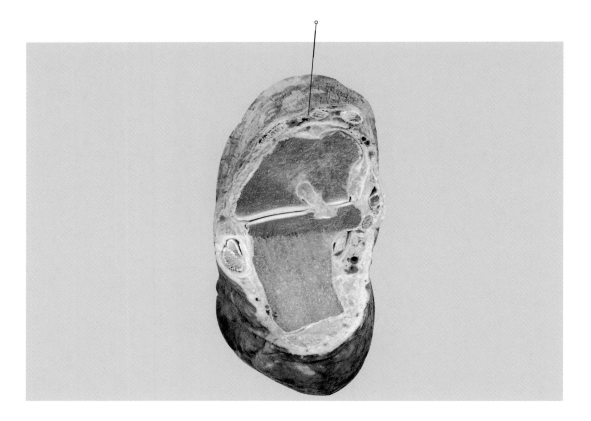

Fig. 5-2 (18) Transverse sectional figure of ST-41 Jiexi (left)

ST-41 Jiexi

Location On the anterior side of the ankle joint, at the midpoint of the transverse crease of the junction between the dorsum of the foot and leg, in the depression between the tendons of the extensor hallucis longus and extensor digitorum longus muscles.

Method Insert perpendicularly 0.5 cun.

Actions Invigorates the channels, alleviates pain, clears Heat, and calms the Spirit.

Indications Headache, nephritis, enteritis, epilepsy, diseases of the ankle joint and its peripheral soft tissue, and foot drop.

Stratified anatomy 1. skin; 2. subcutaneous tissue; 3. tendons of (a) the extensor hallucis longus and (b) extensor digitorum longus muscles; 4. deep peroneal nerve and anterior tibial artery and vein; 5. talus.

Caution The anterior tibial vessels and nerve lie deep to this point.

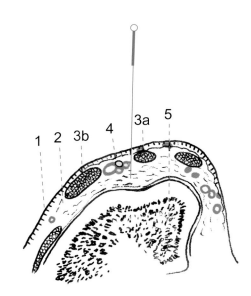

Transverse sectional figure of ST-41 Jiexi (left)

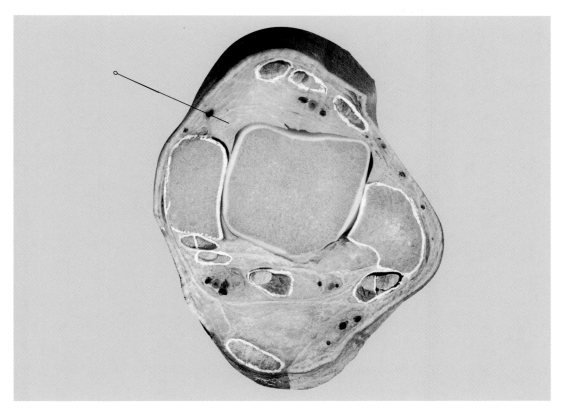

Fig. 5-2 (19) Transverse sectional figure of SP-5 Shangqiu (right)

SP-5 Shangqiu

Location On the medial side of the foot, anterior and inferior to the medial malleolus, at the midpoint between the tip of the medial malleolus and the tuberosity of the navicular bone.

Method Insert perpendicularly 0.2-0.5 cun.

Actions Benefits the Spleen and Stomach and transforms Dampness.

Indications Gastritis, enteritis, dyspepsia, beriberi, edema, and diseases of the ankle joint and its peripheral soft tissue.

Stratified anatomy 1. skin; 2. subcutaneous tissue; 3. triangular ligament; 4. medial malleolus.

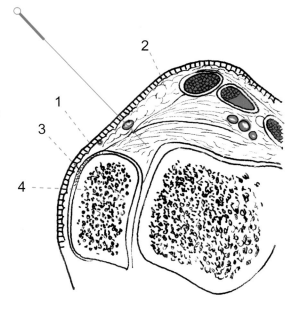

Transverse sectional figure
of SP-5 Shangqiu (right)

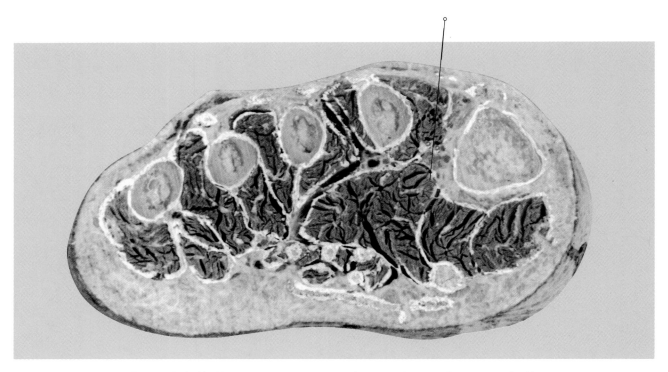

Fig. 5-2 (20) Transverse sectional figure of LR-3 Taichong (left)

LR-3 Taichong

Location On the dorsum of the foot, in the depression distal to the junction of the first and second metatarsal bones.

Method Insert perpendicularly 0.5-1 cun.

Actions Regulates Liver Qi, extinguishes Wind, and regulates and nourishes the Blood.

Indications Headache, vertigo, insomnia, hypertension, hepatitis, mastitis, thrombocytopenia, profuse menstruation, and aching and painful limbs.

Stratified anatomy 1. skin; 2. subcutaneous tissue; 3. tendons of (a) the extensor hallucis longus muscle and (b) the extensor digitorum longus muscle; 4. lateral to the extensor hallucis brevis muscle; 5. deep peroneal nerve and the first dorsal metatarsal artery and vein; 6. the first dorsal interosseous muscle.

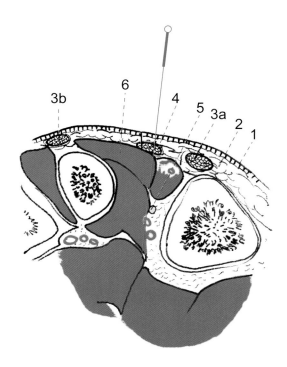

Transverse sectional figure
of LR-3 Taichong (left)

Appendix Computed tomography (CT) scan of acupuncture points

Computed tomography (CT) is a computer-enhanced scanning technique for the analysis of X-ray images. A series of these images is analyzed by computer to generate two-dimensional high-resolution scans representing the anatomical cross-section of the region of the body being imaged. Diagnosis through CT scanning must be derived from the normal sectional anatomical images produced by CT, which should be based on cadaveric sectional anatomical structures. Only through analysis and comparison can a correct diagnosis be made. However, to the author's knowledge, there are currently no reports or books on the sectional anatomy of acupuncture points with CT inside or outside China.

Professor Yan began to study this issue in the Affiliated Hospital of the Medical School attached to Osaka Municipal University in Japan in 1982. He took 157 CT scans of commonly used acupuncture points. This atlas has selected some of these scans to analyze the images and draw sectional figures to indicate the stratified structure of important acupuncture points; these have been labeled with anatomical names to indicate the location of certain important structures.

Fig. 6-1 CT scan of LI-20 Yingxiang and SI-18 Quanliao

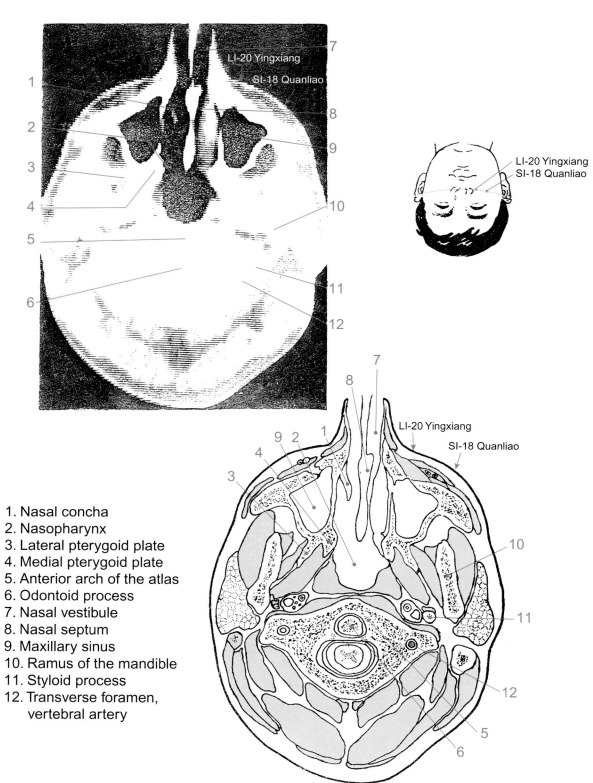

1. Nasal concha
2. Nasopharynx
3. Lateral pterygoid plate
4. Medial pterygoid plate
5. Anterior arch of the atlas
6. Odontoid process
7. Nasal vestibule
8. Nasal septum
9. Maxillary sinus
10. Ramus of the mandible
11. Styloid process
12. Transverse foramen,
    vertebral artery

Fig. 6-2 CT scan of LI-18 Futu and SI-16 Tianchuang

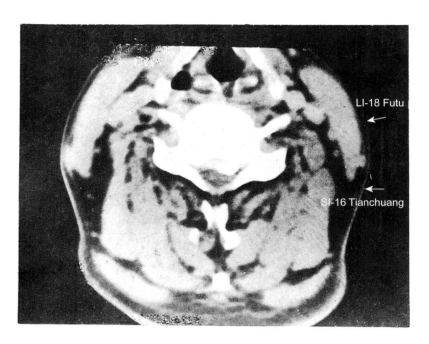

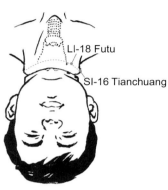

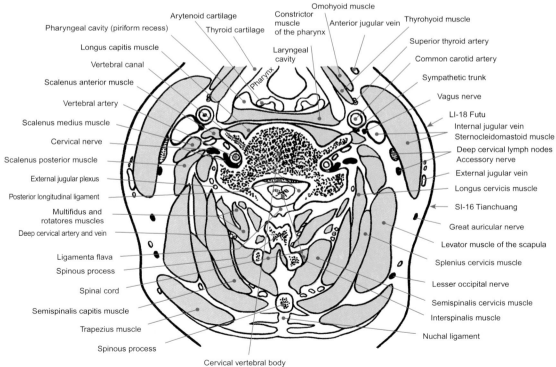

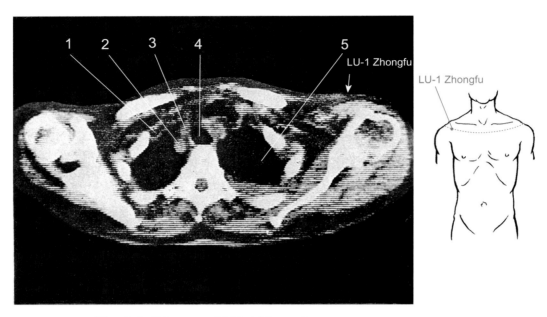

Fig. 6-3 CT scan of LU-1 Zhongfu

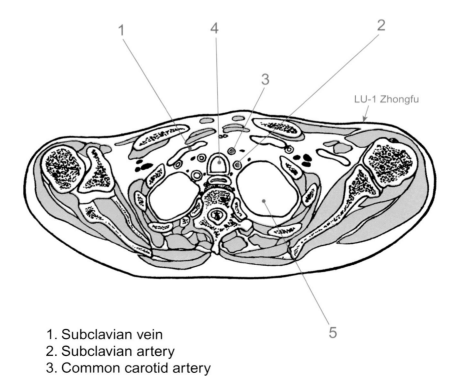

1. Subclavian vein
2. Subclavian artery
3. Common carotid artery
4. Trachea
5. Upper lobe of the right lung

Fig. 6-4 CT scan of LI-4 Hegu

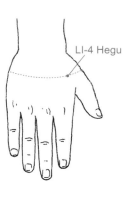

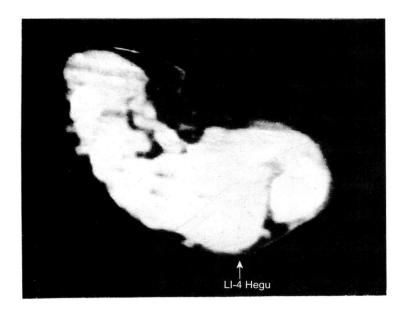

LI-4 Hegu

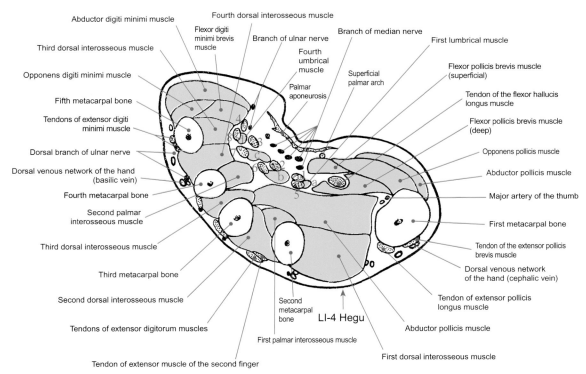

Abductor digiti minimi muscle	Fourth dorsal interosseous muscle
	Flexor digiti minimi brevis muscle
Third dorsal interosseous muscle	Branch of ulnar nerve
	Fourth umbrical muscle
Opponens digiti minimi muscle	Branch of median nerve
	First lumbrical muscle
Fifth metacarpal bone	Superficial palmar arch
Tendons of extensor digiti minimi muscle	Palmar aponeurosis
Dorsal branch of ulnar nerve	Flexor pollicis brevis muscle (superficial)
Dorsal venous network of the hand (basilic vein)	Tendon of the flexor hallucis longus muscle
Fourth metacarpal bone	Flexor pollicis brevis muscle (deep)
Second palmar interosseous muscle	Opponens pollicis muscle
Third dorsal interosseous muscle	Abductor pollicis muscle
Third metacarpal bone	Major artery of the thumb
Second dorsal interosseous muscle	First metacarpal bone
Tendons of extensor digitorum muscles	Tendon of the extensor pollicis brevis muscle
Tendon of extensor muscle of the second finger	Dorsal venous network of the hand (cephalic vein)
	Tendon of extensor pollicis longus muscle
	Abductor pollicis muscle
	First dorsal interosseous muscle

Second metacarpal bone

LI-4 Hegu

First palmar interosseous muscle

1-4. Tendons of the flexor digitorum superficialis muscles
5-8. Tendons of the flexor digitorum profundus muscles
a-d. Lumbrical muscles

Fig. 6-5 CT scan of GB-30 Huantiao

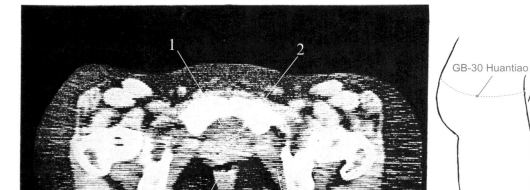

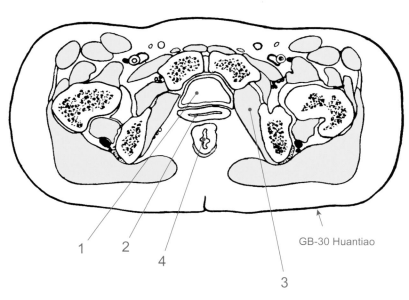

1. Bladder
2. Vagina
3. Obturator internal muscle
4. Rectum

Fig. 6-6 CT scan of ST-36 Zusanli

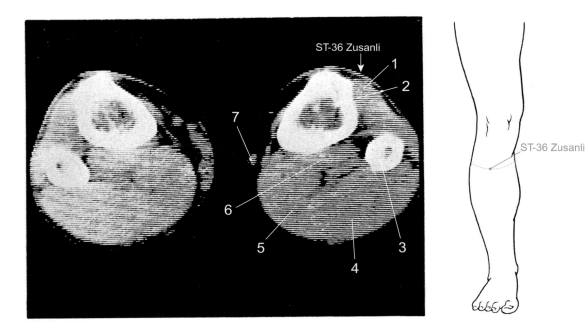

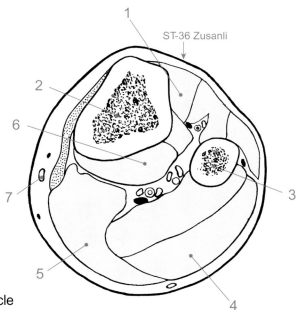

1. Tibialis anterior muscle
2. Tibia
3. Fibula
4. Lateral head of the gastrocnemius muscle
5. Medial head of the gastrocnemius muscle
6. Flexor digitorum longus muscle
7. Long saphenous vein

Index

CLASSIFICATION OF POINTS BY CHANNEL

Lung channel of hand-Taiyin
LU-1 Zhongfu, 3, 7, 178
LU-2 Yunmen, 3, 7, 91
LU-3 Tianfu, 3, 7, 37, 38, 41, 136
LU-4 Xiabai, 3, 7, 37, 38, 41, 136
LU-5 Chize, 3, 7, 37, 38, 41, 43, 136, 137, 141
LU-6 Kongzui, 3, 7, 37, 38, 43, 141
LU-7 Lieque, 3, 7, 37, 40, 43, 44, 147
LU-8 Jingqu, 3, 7, 37, 40, 43, 44
LU-9 Taiyuan, 3, 7, 37, 40, 43, 44, 45, 141
LU-10 Yuji, 3, 7, 37, 37, 40, 45, 152
LU-11 Shaoshang, 3, 7, 38

Large Intestine channel of hand-Yangming
LI-1 Shangyang, 5, 6, 8, 37, 38, 46
LI-2 Erjian, 5, 6, 8, 37, 38, 46
LI-3 Sanjian, 5, 6, 8, 37, 38, 46
LI-4 Hegu, 5, 6, 8, 37, 38, 46, 153, 179
LI-5 Yangxi, 5, 6, 8, 37, 43, 46, 138, 139, 140
LI-6 Pianli, 5, 6, 8, 37, 43
LI-7 Wenliu, 5, 6, 8, 37, 43
LI-8 Xialian, 5, 6, 8, 37, 43, 140
LI-9 Shanglian, 5, 6, 8, 37, 43, 139
LI-10 Shousanli, 5, 6, 8, 37, 43, 138
LI-11 Quchi, 5, 6, 8, 37, 41, 43, 138, 139, 140
LI-12 Zhouliao, 5, 6, 8, 37, 41
LI-13 Shouwuli, 5, 6, 8, 37, 41
LI-14 Binao, 5, 6, 8, 41
LI-15 Jianyu, 5, 6, 8, 135
LI-16 Jugu, 5, 6
LI-17 Tianding, 5, 6, 9, 31, 33, 34, 36
LI-18 Futu, 5, 6, 9, 31, 33, 34, 36, 88, 177
LI-19 Kouheliao, 5, 6, 9, 31, 33, 34
LI-20 Yingxiang, 5, 6, 9, 31, 33, 34, 82, 176

Stomach channel of hand-Jueyin
ST-1 Chengqi, 1, 31, 33, 34, 89
ST-2 Sibai, 1, 31, 33, 34, 82, 89
ST-3 Juliao, 1, 31, 33, 34
ST-4 Dicang, 1, 31, 33, 34, 84
ST-5 Daying, 1, 31, 33, 34
ST-6 Jiache, 33, 34
ST-7 Xiaguan, 33, 34
ST-8 Touwei, 33, 34, 35
ST-9 Renying, 1, 31, 33, 34, 36, 88
ST-10 Shuitu, 1, 31, 33, 34, 36
ST-11 Qishe, 1, 31, 33, 34, 36
ST-12 Quepen, 1, 10, 31, 33, 34, 36
ST-13 Qihu, 1, 10, 19, 23, 70, 71
ST-14 Kufang, 1, 10, 19, 23, 70, 71, 93
ST-15 Wuyi, 1, 10, 19, 23, 70, 71
ST-16 Yingchuang, 1, 10, 19, 23, 70, 71, 96
ST-17 Ruzhong, 1, 10, 19, 23, 70, 71
ST-18 Rugen, 1, 10, 19, 23, 70, 71

ST-19 Burong, 1, 10, 19, 23, 67, 69
ST-20 Chengman, 1, 10, 19, 23, 67, 69
ST-21 Liangmen, 1, 10, 19, 23, 67, 69
ST-22 Guanmen, 1, 10, 19, 23, 67, 69
ST-23 Taiyi, 1, 10, 19, 67, 69
ST-24 Huaroumen, 1, 10, 19, 67, 69
ST-25 Tianshu, 1, 10, 19, 24, 67, 69, 106
ST-26 Wailing, 1, 10, 19, 24, 67, 69
ST-27 Daju, 1, 10, 19, 24, 67, 69
ST-28 Shuidao, 1, 10, 19, 24, 67, 69
ST-29 Guilai, 1, 10, 19, 24, 67, 69
ST-30 Qichong, 1, 10, 19, 24, 67, 69
ST-31 Biguan, 1, 10, 47, 51
ST-32 Futu, 1, 10, 47, 51, 160
ST-33 Yinshi, 1, 10, 47, 51
ST-34 Liangqiu, 1, 10, 47, 51
ST-35 Dubi, 1, 10, 47, 51, 55, 160, 164, 165
ST-36 Zusanli, 1, 10, 47, 55, 164, 165, 166, 181
ST-37 Shangjuxu, 1, 10, 47, 55, 166
ST-38 Tiaokou, 1, 10, 47, 55, 167
ST-39 Xiajuxu, 1, 10, 47, 55
ST-40 Fenglong, 1, 10, 47, 55, 167
ST-41 Jiexi, 1, 10, 47, 55, 57, 172
ST-42 Chongyang, 1, 10, 47, 57
ST-43 Xiangu, 1, 10, 47, 57
ST-44 Neiting, 1, 10, 47, 57
ST-45 Lidui, 1, 10, 47, 57

Spleen channel of foot-Taiyin
SP-1 Yinbai, 3, 11, 49, 56, 58
SP-2 Dadu, 3, 11, 49, 56, 58
SP-3 Taibai, 3, 11, 49, 56, 58
SP-4 Gongsun, 3, 11, 49, 56, 58
SP-5 Shangqiu, 3, 11, 49, 56, 58, 173
SP-6 Sanyinjiao, 3, 11, 49, 56, 170
SP-7 Lougu, 3, 11, 49, 56
SP-8 Diji, 3, 11, 49, 56
SP-9 Yinlingquan, 3, 11, 49, 56
SP-10 Xuehai, 3, 11, 49, 53, 161
SP-11 Jimen, 3, 11, 49, 53
SP-12 Chongmen, 3, 11, 19, 24, 70, 72
SP-13 Fushe, 3, 11, 19, 24, 70, 72
SP-14 Fujie, 3, 11, 19, 24, 70, 72
SP-15 Daheng, 3, 11, 19, 24, 70, 72
SP-16 Fu'ai, 3, 11, 19, 23, 70, 72
SP-17 Shidou, 3, 11, 19, 22, 23
SP-18 Tianxi, 3, 11, 19, 22, 23
SP-19 Xiongxiang, 3, 11, 19, 22, 23
SP-20 Zhourong, 3, 11, 19, 22, 23, 94
SP-21 Dabao, 11, 39

Heart channel of hand-Shaoyin
HT-1 Jiquan, 7, 37, 39, 40, 41, 42
HT-2 Qingling, 7, 37, 40, 41, 42

HT-3 Shaohai, 7, 37, 40, 41, 42, 43, 44
HT-4 Lingdao, 7, 37, 40, 43, 44
HT-5 Tongli, 7, 37, 40, 43, 44, 148
HT-6 Yinxi, 7, 37, 40, 43, 44, 149
HT-7 Shenmen, 7, 37, 40, 43, 44, 45, 148, 149, 150
HT-8 Shaofu, 7, 37, 40, 45
HT-9 Shaochong, 37, 46

Small Intestine channel of hand-Taiyang
SI-1 Shaoze, 4, 12, 37, 38, 44, 46
SI-2 Qiangu, 4, 12, 37, 38, 44, 46
SI-3 Houxi, 4, 12, 37, 38, 44, 46
SI-4 Wangu, 4, 12, 37, 38, 44, 46, 151
SI-5 Yanggu, 4, 12, 37, 38, 43, 46
SI-6 Yanglao, 4, 12, 37, 38, 43
SI-7 Zhizheng, 4, 12, 37, 38, 43
SI-8 Xiaohai, 4, 12, 37, 38, 41, 43
SI-9 Jianzhen, 4, 12, 37, 38, 41
SI-10 Naoshu, 4, 12
SI-11 Tianzong, 4, 12
SI-12 Bingfeng, 4, 12
SI-13 Quyuan, 4, 12
SI-14 Jianwaishu, 4, 12
SI-15 Jianzhongshu, 4, 12
SI-16 Tianchuang, 4, 12, 32, 33, 34, 177
SI-17 Tianrong, 12, 33, 34, 86
SI-18 Quanliao, 12, 33, 34, 176
SI-19 Tinggong, 12, 33, 34

Bladder channel of foot-Taiyang
BL-1 Jingming, 9, 31, 79
BL-2 Cuanzhu, 9, 31, 33, 34
BL-3 Meichong, 9, 33, 34, 35
BL-4 Qucha, 9, 33, 34, 35
BL-5 Wuchu, 9, 33, 34, 35
BL-6 Chengguang, 9, 33, 34, 35
BL-7 Tongtian, 9, 33, 34, 35
BL-8 Luoque, 9, 32, 33, 34, 35
BL-9 Yuzhen, 32, 33, 34
BL-10 Tianzhu, 2, 32, 33, 34
BL-11 Dazhu, 2, 8, 20, 25, 73, 74
BL-12 Fengmen, 2, 8, 20, 25, 73, 74
BL-13 Feishu, 2, 8, 20, 25, 73, 74, 114
BL-14 Jueyinshu, 2, 8, 20, 25, 73, 74, 115
BL-15 Xinshu, 2, 8, 20, 25, 73, 74, 116
BL-16 Dushu, 2, 8, 20, 25, 73, 74, 117
BL-17 Geshu, 2, 8, 20, 25, 73, 74, 118
BL-18 Ganshu, 2, 8, 20, 25, 73, 74, 120
BL-19 Danshu, 2, 8, 20, 25, 73, 74, 121
BL-20 Pishu, 2, 8, 20, 25, 73, 74, 122
BL-21 Weishu, 2, 8, 20, 25, 73, 74, 123
BL-22 Sanjiaoshu, 2, 8, 20, 25, 73, 75, 124
BL-23 Shenshu, 2, 8, 20, 26, 73, 75, 125
BL-24 Qihaishu, 2, 8, 20, 26, 73, 75, 126

BL-25 Dachangshu, 2, 8, 20, 26, 73, 75, 127
BL-26 Guanyuanshu, 2, 8, 20, 26, 73, 75, 128
BL-27 Xiaochangshu, 2, 8, 20, 26, 73, 75
BL-28 Pangguangshu, 2, 8, 20, 26, 73, 75
BL-29 Zhonglüshu, 2, 8, 20, 26, 73, 75
BL-30 Baihuanshu, 2, 8, 20, 26, 73, 75
BL-31 Shangliao, 2, 8, 20, 26, 129
BL-32 Ciliao, 2, 8, 20, 26, 130
BL-33 Zhongliao, 2, 8, 20, 26, 131
BL-34 Xialiao, 2, 8, 20, 26, 132
BL-35 Huiyang, 2, 8, 20, 26
BL-36 Chengfu, 2, 8, 48, 52, 157, 158
BL-37 Yinmen, 2, 8, 48, 52, 158
BL-38 Fuxi, 2, 8, 48, 52
BL-39 Weiyang, 2, 8, 48, 52, 55
BL-40 Weizhong, 2, 4, 8, 48, 52, 55, 56
BL-41 Fufen, 4, 8, 20, 25, 76, 77
BL-42 Pohu, 4, 8, 20, 25, 76, 77
BL-43 Gaohuang, 4, 8, 20, 25, 76, 77
BL-44 Shentang, 4, 8, 20, 25, 76, 77
BL-45 Yixi, 4, 8, 20, 25, 76, 77
BL-46 Geguan, 4, 8, 20, 25, 76, 77
BL-47 Hunmen, 4, 8, 20, 25, 76, 77
BL-48 Yanggang, 4, 8, 20, 25, 76, 77
BL-49 Yishe, 4, 8, 20, 25, 76, 77
BL-50 Weicang, 4, 8, 20, 25, 76, 77
BL-51 Huangmen, 4, 8, 20, 25, 76, 78
BL-52 Zhishi, 4, 8, 20, 26, 76, 78
BL-53 Baohuang, 4, 8, 20, 26, 76, 78
BL-54 Zhibian, 4, 8, 20, 26, 76, 78
BL-55 Heyang, 4, 8, 48, 55
BL-56 Chengjin, 4, 8, 48, 55
BL-57 Chengshan, 4, 8, 48, 55
BL-58 Feiyang, 4, 8, 48, 50, 55, 56
BL-59 Fuyang, 4, 8, 48, 50, 55, 56
BL-60 Kunlun, 4, 8, 48, 50, 56, 58
BL-61 Pucan, 4, 8, 48, 50, 56, 58
BL-62 Shenmai, 4, 8, 48, 50, 56, 58
BL-63 Jinmen, 4, 8, 48, 50, 56, 58
BL-64 Jinggu, 4, 8, 48, 50, 56, 58
BL-65 Shugu, 4, 8, 48, 50, 56, 58
BL-66 Zutonggu, 4, 8, 48, 50, 56, 58
BL-67 Zhiyin, 4, 8, 48, 50, 56, 58

Kidney channel of foot-Shaoyin
KI-1 Yongquan, 57
KI-2 Rangu, 13, 49, 56, 58
KI-3 Taixi, 13, 49, 56, 58, 168, 171
KI-4 Dazhong, 13, 49, 56, 58
KI-5 Shuiquan, 13, 49, 56, 58
KI-6 Zhaohai, 13, 49, 56, 58
KI-7 Fuliu, 13, 49, 56, 171
KI-8 Jiaoxin, 13, 49, 56
KI-9 Zhubin, 13, 49, 56, 168
KI-10 Yingu, 13, 48, 49, 53, 55, 56, 168
KI-11 Henggu, 3, 13, 19, 24, 64, 66
KI-12 Dahe, 3, 13, 19, 24, 64, 66
KI-13 Qixue, 3, 13, 19, 24, 64, 66
KI-14 Siman, 3, 13, 19, 24, 64, 66

KI-15 Zhongzhu, 3, 13, 19, 24, 64, 66
KI-16 Huangshu, 3, 13, 19, 24, 64, 66
KI-17 Shangqu, 3, 13, 19, 23, 64, 65
KI-18 Shiguan, 3, 13, 19, 23, 64, 65
KI-19 Yindu, 3, 13, 19, 23, 64, 65
KI-20 Futonggu, 3, 13, 19, 23, 64, 65
KI-21 Youmen, 3, 13, 19, 23, 64, 65
KI-22 Bulang, 3, 13, 19, 23, 67, 68, 98
KI-23 Shenfeng, 3, 13, 19, 23, 67, 68
KI-24 Lingxu, 3, 13, 19, 23, 67, 68
KI-25 Shencang, 3, 13, 19, 23, 67, 68, 95
KI-26 Yuzhong, 3, 13, 19, 23, 67, 68
KI-27 Shufu, 3, 13, 19, 23, 67, 68

Pericardium channel of foot-Yangming
PC-1 Tianchi, 1, 10
PC-2 Tianquan, 1, 10, 37, 40, 41, 42
PC-3 Quze, 1, 10, 37, 40, 41, 42, 43, 44, 143
PC-4 Ximen, 1, 10, 37, 40, 43, 44, 143
PC-5 Jianshi, 1, 10, 37, 40, 43, 44, 145
PC-6 Neiguan, 1, 10, 37, 40, 43, 44, 146
PC-7 Daling, 1, 10, 37, 40, 43, 44, 45, 143, 144
PC-8 Laogong, 1, 10, 37, 40, 45, 154
PC-9 Zhongchong, 1, 10, 37, 40, 45

Triple Burner channel of hand-Shaoyang
TB-1 Guanchong, 2, 12, 37, 46
TB-2 Yemen, 2, 12, 37, 46
TB-3 Zhongzhu, 2, 12, 37, 46
TB-4 Yangchi, 2, 12, 37, 43, 46
TB-5 Waiguan, 2, 12, 37, 43
TB-6 Zhigou, 2, 12, 37, 43
TB-7 Huizong, 2, 12, 37, 43
TB-8 Sanyangluo, 2, 12, 37, 43
TB-9 Sidu, 2, 12, 37, 43
TB-10 Tianjing, 2, 12, 37, 41
TB-11 Qinglengyuan, 2, 12, 37, 41
TB-12 Xiaoluo, 2, 12, 37, 41
TB-13 Naohui, 2, 12, 37, 41
TB-14 Jianliao, 2, 12, 37, 41
TB-15 Tianliao, 2
TB-16 Tianyou, 32, 33, 34
TB-17 Yifeng, 32, 33, 34, 83
TB-18 Chimai, 32, 33, 34
TB-19 Luxi, 32, 33, 34
TB-20 Jiaosun, 32, 33, 34
TB-21 Ermen, 33, 34
TB-22 Erheliao, 33, 34
TB-23 Sizhukong, 31, 33, 34

Gallbladder channel of foot-Shaoyang
GB-1 Tongziliao, 15, 31, 33, 34
GB-2 Tinghui, 15, 33, 34
GB-3 Shangguan, 15, 33, 34, 80
GB-4 Hanyan, 15, 33, 34
GB-5 Xuanlu, 15, 33, 34
GB-6 Xuanli, 15, 33, 34
GB-7 Qubin, 15, 33, 34
GB-8 Shuaigu, 15, 33, 34

GB-9 Tianchong, 15, 32, 33, 34
GB-10 Fubai, 15, 32, 33, 34
GB-11 Touqiaoyin, 15, 32, 33, 34
GB-12 Wangu, 15, 32, 33, 34
GB-13 Benshen, 15, 33, 34, 35
GB-14 Yangbai, 15, 31, 33, 34, 35
GB-15 Toulinqi, 15, 33, 34, 35
GB-16 Muchuang, 15, 33, 34, 35
GB-17 Zhengying, 15, 33, 34, 35
GB-18 Chengling, 15, 32, 33, 34, 35
GB-19 Naokong, 15, 32, 33, 34
GB-20 Fengchi, 15, 32, 33, 34, 85
GB-21 Jianjing, 32
GB-22 Yuanye, 5, 6, 14, 21, 27, 39
GB-23 Zhejin, 5, 6, 14, 21, 27, 39
GB-24 Riyue, 5, 6, 14, 21, 22, 27
GB-25 Jingmen, 5, 6, 14, 21, 22, 26, 28
GB-26 Daimai, 5, 6, 14, 21, 22, 28
GB-27 Wushu, 14, 21, 22
GB-28 Weidao, 14, 21, 22
GB-29 Juliao, 14, 50, 54
GB-30 Huantiao, 5, 6, 14, 26, 50, 54, 155, 180
GB-31 Fengshi, 5, 6, 14, 50, 54, 159
GB-32 Zhongdu, 5, 6, 14, 50, 54
GB-33 Xiyangguan, 5, 6, 14, 50, 54, 56
GB-34 Yanglingquan, 5, 6, 14, 50, 56, 162, 163
GB-35 Yangjiao, 5, 6, 14, 50, 56
GB-36 Waiqiu, 5, 6, 14, 48, 50, 56
GB-37 Guangming, 5, 6, 14, 50, 56, 169
GB-38 Yangfu, 5, 6, 14, 50, 56
GB-39 Xuanzhong, 5, 6, 14, 50, 56
GB-40 Qiuxu, 5, 6, 14, 50, 56, 57, 58
GB-41 Zulinqi, 5, 6, 14, 50, 56, 57, 58
GB-42 Diwuhui, 5, 6, 14, 50, 56, 57, 58
GB-43 Xiaxi, 5, 6, 14, 50, 56, 57, 58
GB-44 Zuqiaoyin, 5, 6, 14, 50, 56, 57, 58

Liver channel of foot-Jueyin
LR-1 Dadun, 11, 49, 56, 57, 58
LR-2 Xingjian, 11, 49, 56, 57, 58
LR-3 Taichong, 11, 49, 56, 57, 58, 174
LR-4 Zhongfeng, 11, 49, 56, 57, 58
LR-5 Ligou, 11, 49, 56
LR-6 Zhongdu, 11, 49, 56
LR-7 Xiguan, 11, 49, 56
LR-8 Ququan, 11, 49, 53
LR-9 Yinbao, 11, 49, 53
LR-10 Zuwuli, 11, 49, 53
LR-11 Yinlian, 11, 49, 53, 156
LR-12 Jimai, 11
LR-13 Zhangmen, 11, 21, 22, 28
LR-14 Qimen, 11, 21, 22, 27

Governor vessel
GV-1 Changqiang, 2, 4, 16, 20, 26, 30, 61, 63, 133
GV-2 Yaoshu, 2, 4, 16, 20, 26, 61, 63
GV-3 Yaoyangguan, 2, 4, 16, 20, 26, 61, 63
GV-4 Mingmen 2, 4, 16, 20, 26, 61, 63
GV-5 Xuanshu, 2, 4, 16, 20, 25, 61, 63
GV-6 Jizhong, 2, 4, 16, 20, 25, 61, 63

GV-7 Zhongshu, 2, 4, 16, 20, 25, 61, 63
GV-8 Jinsuo, 2, 4, 16, 20, 25, 61, 63
GV-9 Zhiyang, 2, 4, 16, 20, 25, 61, 62
GV-10 Lingtai, 2, 4, 16, 20, 25, 61, 62
GV-11 Shendao, 2, 4, 16, 20, 25, 61, 62
GV-12 Shenzhu, 2, 4, 16, 20, 25, 61, 62
GV-13 Taodao, 2, 4, 16, 20, 25, 61, 62
GV-14 Dazhui, 2, 4, 16, 20, 25, 61, 62, 113
GV-15 Yamen, 2, 16, 32, 61, 62
GV-16 Fengfu, 32, 61, 62, 85
GV-17 Naohu, 32, 61, 62
GV-18 Qiangjian, 32, 61, 62
GV-19 Houding, 32, 35, 61, 62
GV-20 Baihui, 32, 35, 61, 62
GV-21 Qianding, 35, 61, 62
GV-22 Xinhui, 17, 35, 61, 62
GV-23 Shangxing, 17, 35, 61, 62
GV-24 Shenting, 17, 35, 61, 62
GV-25 Suliao, 17, 31, 33, 34, 61, 62
GV-26 Shuigou, 17, 31, 33, 34, 61, 62
GV-27 Duiduan, 17, 31, 33, 34, 61, 62

Conception vessel
CV-1 Huiyin, 30
CV-2 Qugu, 1, 3, 13, 19, 24, 61, 63, 112, 156
CV-3 Zhongji, 1, 3, 13, 19, 24, 61, 63, 111
CV-4 Guanyuan, 1, 3, 13, 19, 24, 61, 63, 110
CV-5 Shimen, 1, 3, 13, 19, 24, 61, 63, 109
CV-6 Qihai, 1, 3, 13, 19, 24, 61, 63, 108
CV-7 Yinjiao, 1, 3, 13, 19, 24, 61, 63, 107

CV-8 Shenque, 1, 3, 13, 19, 24, 61, 63
CV-9 Shuifen, 1, 3, 13, 19, 23, 61, 63, 105
CV-10 Xiawan, 1, 3, 13, 19, 23, 61, 63, 104
CV-11 Jianli, 1, 3, 13, 19, 23, 61, 63, 103
CV-12 Zhongwan, 1, 3, 13, 19, 23, 61, 63, 102
CV-13 Shangwan, 1, 3, 13, 19, 23, 61, 63, 101
CV-14 Juque, 1, 3, 13, 19, 23, 61, 63, 100
CV-15 Jiuwei, 1, 3, 13, 19, 23, 61, 63, 99
CV-16 Zhongting, 1, 3, 13, 19, 23, 61, 62, 98
CV-17 Danzhong, 1, 3, 13, 19, 23, 61, 62, 97
CV-18 Yutang, 1, 3, 13, 19, 23, 61, 62, 96, 97
CV-19 Zigong, 1, 3, 13, 19, 23, 61, 62, 95
CV-20 Huagai, 1, 3, 13, 19, 23, 61, 62, 93
CV-21 Xuanji, 1, 3, 13, 19, 23, 61, 62
CV-22 Tiantu, 1, 3, 13, 23, 31, 33, 34, 36, 61, 62, 92
CV-23 Lianquan, 1, 3, 13, 31, 33, 34, 36, 61, 62, 87
CV-24 Chengjiang, 1, 3, 13, 31, 33, 34, 61, 62

Extra points
EX-B-1 Dingchuan, 25
EX-B-3 Weiwanxiashu (Weiguanxiashu), 25, 119
EX-B-4 Pigen, 25
EX-B-6 Yaoyi, 26
EX-B-7 Yaoyan, 26
EX-B-8 Shiqizhui, 2, 26
EX-B-9 Yaoqi, 26
EX-CA-1 Zigong, 29
EX-HN-3 Yintang, 31, 35
EX-HN-4 Yuyao, 31

EX-HN-7 Qiuhou, 31
EX-HN-14 Yiming, 33, 34, 83
EX-LE-1 Kuangu, 47, 51
EX-LE-2 Heding, 47, 51
EX-LE-3 Baichongwo, 49
EX-LE-4 Neixiyan, 47, 51
EX-LE-6 Dannang, 5, 50, 56, 163
EX-LE-7 Lanwei, 47, 55, 165
EX-LE-8 Neihuaijian, 49, 56
EX-LE-9 Waihuaijian, 48, 50, 56, 58
EX-LE-10 Bafeng, 57
EX-LE-11 Duyin, 57
EX-LE-12 Qiduan, 57
EX-UE-1 Zhoujian, 41, 43
EX-UE-2 Erbai, 43, 44, 144
EX-UE-3 Zhongquan, 46
EX-UE-4 Zhongkui, 46
EX-UE-5 Dagukong, 46
EX-UE-6 Xiaogukong, 46
EX-UE-7 Yaotongdian, 46
EX-UE-8 Wailaogong, 46
EX-UE-9 Baxie, 46
EX-UE-10 Sifeng, 45
EX-UE-11 Shixuan, 45
Bitong, 31, 81, 82
Bizhong, 37, 40, 43, 142
Luozhen, 46

Ear acupuncture points
Anterior lateral side of the auricle, 59
Dorsum of the auricle, 60

CLASSIFICATION OF POINTS IN ALPHABETICAL ORDER

Anterior lateral side of the auricle, 59

Bafeng EX-LE-10, 57
Baichongwo EX-LE-3, 49
Baihuanshu BL-30, 2, 8, 20, 26, 73, 75
Baihui GV-20, 32, 35, 61, 62
Baohuang BL-53, 4, 8, 20, 26, 76, 78
Baxie EX-UE-9, 46
Benshen GB-13, 15, 33, 34, 35
Biguan ST-31, 1, 10, 47, 51
Binao LI-14, 5, 6, 8, 41
Bingfeng SI-12, 4, 12
Bitong, 31, 81, 82
Bizhong, 37, 40, 43, 142
Bulang KI-22, 3, 13, 19, 23, 67, 68, 98
Burong ST-19, 1, 10, 19, 23, 67, 69

Changqiang GV-1, 2, 4, 16, 20, 26, 30, 61, 63, 133
Chengfu BL-36, 2, 8, 48, 52, 157, 158
Chengguang BL-6, 9, 33, 34, 35

Chengjiang CV-24, 1, 3, 13, 31, 33, 34, 61, 62
Chengjin BL-56, 4, 8, 48, 55
Chengling GB-18, 15, 32, 33, 34, 35
Chengman ST-20, 1, 10, 19, 23, 67, 69
Chengqi ST-1, 1, 31, 33, 34, 89
Chengshan BL-57, 4, 8, 48, 55
Chimai TB-18, 32, 33, 34
Chize LU-5, 3, 7, 37, 38, 41, 43, 136, 137, 141
Chongmen SP-12, 3, 11, 19, 24, 70, 72
Chongyang ST-42, 1, 10, 47, 57
Ciliao BL-32, 2, 8, 20, 26, 130
Cuanzhu BL-2, 9, 31, 33, 34

Dabao SP-21, 11, 39
Dachangshu BL-25, 2, 8, 20, 26, 73, 75, 127
Dadu SP-2, 3, 11, 49, 56, 58
Dadun LR-1, 11, 49, 56, 57, 58
Dagukong EX-UE-5, 46
Dahe KI-12, 3, 13, 19, 24, 64, 66
Daheng SP-15, 3, 11, 19, 24, 70, 72

Daimai GB-26, 5, 6, 14, 21, 22, 28
Daju ST-27, 1, 10, 19, 24, 67, 69
Daling PC-7, 1, 10, 37, 40, 43, 44, 45, 143, 144
Dannang EX-LE-6, 5, 50, 56, 163
Danshu BL-19, 2, 8, 20, 25, 73, 74, 121
Danzhong CV-17, 1, 3, 13, 19, 23, 61, 62, 97
Daying ST-5, 1, 31, 33, 34
Dazhong KI-4, 13, 49, 56, 58
Dazhu BL-11, 2, 8, 20, 25, 73, 74
Dazhui GV-14, 2, 4, 16, 20, 25, 61, 62, 113
Dicang ST-4, 1, 31, 33, 34, 84
Diji SP-8, 3, 11, 49, 56
Dingchuan EX-B-1, 25
Diwuhui GB-42, 5, 6, 14, 50, 56, 57, 58
Dorsum of the auricle, 60
Dubi ST-35, 1, 10, 47, 51, 55, 160, 164, 165
Duiduan GV-27, 17, 31, 33, 34, 61, 62
Dushu BL-16, 2, 8, 20, 25, 73, 74, 117
Duyin EX-LE-11, 57

Erbai EX-UE-2, 43, 44, 144

Erheliao TB-22, 33, 34
Erjian LI-2, 5, 6, 8, 37, 38, 46
Ermen TB-21, 33, 34

Feishu BL-13, 2, 8, 20, 25, 73, 74, 114
Feiyang BL-58, 4, 8, 48, 50, 55, 56
Fengchi GB-20, 15, 32, 33, 34, 85
Fengfu GV-16, 32, 61, 62, 85
Fenglong ST-40, 1, 10, 47, 55, 167
Fengmen BL-12, 2, 8, 20, 25, 73, 74
Fengshi GB-31, 5, 6, 14, 50, 54, 159
Fu'ai SP-16, 3, 11, 19, 23, 70, 72
Fubai GB-10, 15, 32, 33, 34
Fufen BL-41, 4, 8, 20, 25, 76, 77
Fujie SP-14, 3, 11, 19, 24, 70, 72
Fuliu KI-7, 13, 49, 56, 171
Fushe SP-13, 3, 11, 19, 24, 70, 72
Futonggu KI-20, 3, 13, 19, 23, 64, 65
Futu LI-18, 5, 6, 9, 31, 33, 34, 36, 88, 177
Futu ST-32, 1, 10, 47, 51, 160
Fuxi BL-38, 2, 8, 48, 52
Fuyang BL-59, 4, 8, 48, 50, 55, 56

Ganshu BL-18, 2, 8, 20, 25, 73, 74, 120
Gaohuang BL-43, 4, 8, 20, 25, 76, 77
Geguan BL-46, 4, 8, 20, 25, 76, 77
Geshu BL-17, 2, 8, 20, 25, 73, 74, 118
Gongsun SP-4, 3, 11, 49, 56, 58
Guanchong TB-1, 2, 12, 37, 46
Guangming GB-37, 5, 6, 14, 50, 56, 169
Guanmen ST-22, 1, 10, 19, 23, 67, 69
Guanyuan CV-4, 1, 3, 13, 19, 24, 61, 63, 110
Guanyuanshu BL-26, 2, 8, 20, 26, 73, 75, 128
Guilai ST-29, 1, 10, 19, 24, 67, 69

Hanyan GB-4, 15, 33, 34
Heding EX-LE-2, 47, 51
Hegu LI-4, 5, 6, 8, 37, 38, 46, 153, 179
Henggu KI-11, 3, 13, 19, 24, 64, 66
Heyang BL-55, 4, 8, 48, 55
Houding GV-19, 32, 35, 61, 62
Houxi SI-3, 4, 12, 37, 38, 44, 46
Huagai CV-20, 1, 3, 13, 19, 23, 61, 62, 93
Huangmen BL-51, 4, 8, 20, 25, 76, 78
Huangshu KI-16, 3, 13, 19, 24, 64, 66
Huantiao GB-30, 5, 6, 14, 26, 50, 54, 155, 180
Huaroumen ST-24, 1, 10, 19, 67, 69
Huiyang BL-35, 2, 8, 20, 26
Huiyin CV-1, 30
Huizong TB-7, 2, 12, 37, 43
Hunmen BL-47, 4, 8, 20, 25, 76, 77

Jiache ST-6, 33, 34
Jianjing GB-21, 32
Jianli CV-11, 1, 3, 13, 19, 23, 61, 63, 103
Jianliao TB-14, 2, 12, 37, 41
Jianshi PC-5, 1, 10, 37, 40, 43, 44, 145
Jianwaishu SI-14, 4, 12
Jianyu LI-15, 5, 6, 8, 135

Jianzhen SI-9, 4, 12, 37, 38, 41
Jianzhongshu SI-15, 4, 12
Jiaosun TB-20, 32, 33, 34
Jiaoxin KI-8, 13, 49, 56
Jiexi ST-41, 1, 10, 47, 55, 57, 172
Jimai LR-12, 11
Jimen SP-11, 3, 11, 49, 53
Jinggu BL-64, 4, 8, 48, 50, 56, 58
Jingmen GB-25, 5, 6, 14, 21, 22, 26, 28
Jingming BL-1, 9, 31, 79
Jingqu LU-8, 3, 7, 37, 40, 43, 44
Jinmen BL-63, 4, 8, 48, 50, 56, 58
Jinsuo GV-8, 2, 4, 16, 20, 25, 61, 63
Jiquan HT-1, 7, 37, 39, 40, 41, 42
Jiuwei CV-15, 1, 3, 13, 19, 23, 61, 63, 99
Jizhong GV-6, 2, 4, 16, 20, 25, 61, 63
Jueyinshu BL-14, 2, 8, 20, 25, 73, 74, 115
Jugu LI-16, 5, 6
Juliao GB-29, 14, 50, 54
Juliao ST-3, 1, 31, 33, 34
Juque CV-14, 1, 3, 13, 19, 23, 61, 63, 100

Kongzui LU-6, 3, 7, 37, 38, 43, 141
Kouheliao LI-19, 5, 6, 9, 31, 33, 34
Kuangu EX-LE-1, 47, 51
Kufang ST-14, 1, 10, 19, 23, 70, 71, 93
Kunlun BL-60, 4, 8, 48, 50, 56, 58

Lanwei EX-LE-7, 47, 55, 165
Laogong PC-8, 1, 10, 37, 40, 45, 154
Liangmen ST-21, 1, 10, 19, 23, 67, 69
Liangqiu ST-34, 1, 10, 47, 51
Lianquan CV-23, 1, 3, 13, 31, 33, 34, 36, 61, 62, 87
Lidui ST-45, 1, 10, 47, 57
Lieque LU-7, 3, 7, 37, 40, 43, 44, 147
Ligou LR-5, 11, 49, 56
Lingdao HT-4, 7, 37, 40, 43, 44
Lingtai GV-10, 2, 4, 16, 20, 25, 61, 62
Lingxu KI-24, 3, 13, 19, 23, 67, 68
Lougu SP-7, 3, 11, 49, 56
Luoque BL-8, 9, 32, 33, 34, 35
Luozhen, 46
Luxi TB-19, 32, 33, 34

Meichong BL-3, 9, 33, 34, 35
Mingmen GV-4, 2, 4, 16, 20, 26, 61, 63
Muchuang GB-16, 15, 33, 34, 35

Naohu GV-17, 32, 61, 62
Naohui TB-13, 2, 12, 37, 41
Naokong GB-19, 15, 32, 33, 34
Naoshu SI-10, 4, 12
Neiguan PC-6, 1, 10, 37, 40, 43, 44, 146
Neihuaijian EX-LE-8, 49, 56
Neiting ST-44, 1, 10, 47, 57
Neixiyan EX-LE-4, 47, 51

Pangguangshu BL-28, 2, 8, 20, 26, 73, 75
Pianli LI-6, 5, 6, 8, 37, 43

Pigen EX-B-4, 25
Pishu BL-20, 2, 8, 20, 25, 73, 74, 122
Pohu BL-42, 4, 8, 20, 25, 76, 77
Pucan BL-61, 4, 8, 48, 50, 56, 58

Qianding GV-21, 35, 61, 62
Qiangjian GV-18, 32, 61, 62
Qiangu SI-2, 4, 12, 37, 38, 44, 46
Qichong ST-30, 1, 10, 19, 24, 67, 69
Qiduan EX-LE-12, 57
Qihai CV-6, 1, 3, 13, 19, 24, 61, 63, 108
Qihaishu BL-24, 2, 8, 20, 26, 73, 75, 126
Qihu ST-13, 1, 10, 19, 23, 70, 71
Qimen LR-14, 11, 21, 22, 27
Qinglengyuan TB-11, 2, 12, 37, 41
Qingling HT-2, 7, 37, 40, 41, 42
Qishe ST-11, 1, 31, 33, 34, 36
Qiuhou EX-HN-7, 31
Qiuxu GB-40, 5, 6, 14, 50, 56, 57, 58
Qixue KI-13, 3, 13, 19, 24, 64, 66
Quanliao SI-18, 12, 33, 34, 176
Qubin GB-7, 15, 33, 34
Qucha BL-4, 9, 33, 34, 35
Quchi LI-11, 5, 6, 8, 37, 41, 43, 138, 139, 140
Quepen ST-12, 1, 10, 31, 33, 34, 36
Qugu CV-2, 1, 3, 13, 19, 24, 61, 63, 112, 156
Ququan LR-8, 11, 49, 53
Quyuan SI-13, 4, 12
Quze PC-3, 1, 10, 37, 40, 41, 42, 43, 44, 143

Rangu KI-2, 13, 49, 56, 58
Renying ST-9, 1, 31, 33, 34, 36, 88
Riyue GB-24, 5, 6, 14, 21, 22, 27
Rugen ST-18, 1, 10, 19, 23, 70, 71
Ruzhong ST-17, 1, 10, 19, 23, 70, 71

Sanjian LI-3, 5, 6, 8, 37, 38, 46
Sanjiaoshu BL-22, 2, 8, 20, 25, 73, 75, 124
Sanyangluo TB-8, 2, 12, 37, 43
Sanyinjiao SP-6, 3, 11, 49, 56, 170
Shangguan GB-3, 15, 33, 34, 80
Shangjuxu ST-37, 1, 10, 47, 55, 166
Shanglian LI-9, 5, 6, 8, 37, 43, 139
Shangliao BL-31, 2, 8, 20, 26, 129
Shangqiu SP-5, 3, 11, 49, 56, 58, 173
Shangqu KI-17, 3, 13, 19, 23, 64, 65
Shangwan CV-13, 1, 3, 13, 19, 23, 61, 63, 101
Shangxing GV-23, 17, 35, 61, 62
Shangyang LI-1, 5, 6, 8, 37, 38, 46
Shaochong HT-9, 37, 46
Shaofu HT-8, 7, 37, 40, 45
Shaohai HT-3, 7, 37, 40, 41, 42, 43, 44
Shaoshang LU-11, 3, 7, 38
Shaoze SI-1, 4, 12, 37, 38, 44, 46
Shencang KI-25, 3, 13, 19, 23, 67, 68, 95
Shendao GV-11, 2, 4, 16, 20, 25, 61, 62
Shenfeng KI-23, 3, 13, 19, 23, 67, 68
Shenmai BL-62, 4, 8, 48, 50, 56, 58
Shenmen HT-7, 7, 37, 40, 43, 44, 45, 148, 149,

Shenque CV-8, 1, 3, 13, 19, 24, 61, 63
Shenshu BL-23, 2, 8, 20, 26, 73, 75, 125
Shentang BL-44, 4, 8, 20, 25, 76, 77
Shenting GV-24, 17, 35, 61, 62
Shenzhu GV-12, 2, 4, 16, 20, 25, 61, 62
Shidou SP-17, 3, 11, 19, 22, 23
Shiguan KI-18, 3, 13, 19, 23, 64, 65
Shimen CV-5, 1, 3, 13, 19, 24, 61, 63, 109
Shiqizhui EX-B-8, 2, 26
Shixuan EX-UE-11, 45
Shousanli LI-10, 5, 6, 8, 37, 43, 138
Shouwuli LI-13, 5, 6, 8, 37, 41
Shuaigu GB-8, 15, 33, 34
Shufu KI-27, 3, 13, 19, 23, 67, 68
Shugu BL-65, 4, 8, 48, 50, 56, 58
Shuidao ST-28, 1, 10, 19, 24, 67, 69
Shuifen CV-9, 1, 3, 13, 19, 23, 61, 63, 105
Shuigou GV-26, 17, 31, 33, 34, 61, 62
Shuiquan KI-5, 13, 49, 56, 58
Shuitu ST-10, 1, 31, 33, 34, 36
Sibai ST-2, 1, 31, 33, 34, 82, 89
Sidu TB-9, 2, 12, 37, 43
Sifeng EX-UE-10, 45
Siman KI-14, 3, 13, 19, 24, 64, 66
Sizhukong TB-23, 31, 33, 34
Suliao GV-25, 17, 31, 33, 34, 61, 62

Taibai SP-3, 3, 11, 49, 56, 58
Taichong LR-3, 11, 49, 56, 57, 58, 174
Taixi KI-3, 13, 49, 56, 58, 168, 171
Taiyi ST-23, 1, 10, 19, 67, 69
Taiyuan LU-9, 3, 7, 37, 40, 43, 44, 45, 141
Taodao GV-13, 2, 4, 16, 20, 25, 61, 62
Tianchi PC-1, 1, 10
Tianchong GB-9, 15, 32, 33, 34
Tianchuang SI-16, 4, 12, 32, 33, 34, 177
Tianding LI-17, 5, 6, 9, 31, 33, 34, 36
Tianfu LU-3, 3, 7, 37, 38, 41, 136
Tianjing TB-10, 2, 12, 37, 41
Tianliao TB-15, 2
Tianquan PC-2, 1, 10, 37, 40, 41, 42
Tianrong SI-17, 12, 33, 34, 86
Tianshu ST-25, 1, 10, 19, 24, 67, 69, 106
Tiantu CV-22, 1, 3, 13, 23, 31, 33, 34, 36, 61, 62, 92
Tianxi SP-18, 3, 11, 19, 22, 23
Tianyou TB-16, 32, 33, 34
Tianzhu BL-10, 2, 32, 33, 34
Tianzong SI-11, 4, 12
Tiaokou ST-38, 1, 10, 47, 55, 167
Tinggong SI-19, 12, 33, 34
Tinghui GB-2, 15, 33, 34
Tongli HT-5, 7, 37, 40, 43, 44, 148
Tongtian BL-7, 9, 33, 34, 35
Tongziliao GB-1, 15, 31, 33, 34
Toulinqi GB-15, 15, 33, 34, 35
Touqiaoyin GB-11, 15, 32, 33, 34
Touwei ST-8, 33, 34, 35

Waiguan TB-5, 2, 12, 37, 43

Waihuaijian EX-LE-9, 48, 50, 56, 58
Wailaogong EX-UE-8, 46
Wailing ST-26, 1, 10, 19, 24, 67, 69
Waiqiu GB-36, 5, 6, 14, 48, 50, 56
Wangu GB-12, 15, 32, 33, 34
Wangu SI-4, 4, 12, 37, 38, 44, 46, 151
Weicang BL-50, 4, 8, 20, 25, 76, 77
Weidao GB-28, 14, 21, 22
Weishu BL-21, 2, 8, 20, 25, 73, 74, 123
Weiwanxiashu (Weiguanxiashu) EX-B-3, 25, 119
Weiyang BL-39, 2, 8, 48, 52, 55
Weizhong BL-40, 2, 4, 8, 48, 52, 55, 56
Wenliu LI-7, 5, 6, 8, 37, 43
Wuchu BL-5, 9, 33, 34, 35
Wushu GB-27, 14, 21, 22
Wuyi ST-15, 1, 10, 19, 23, 70, 71

Xiabai LU-4, 3, 7, 37, 38, 41, 136
Xiaguan ST-7, 33, 34
Xiajuxu ST-39, 1, 10, 47, 55
Xialian LI-8, 5, 6, 8, 37, 43, 140
Xialiao BL-34, 2, 8, 20, 26, 132
Xiangu ST-43, 1, 10, 47, 57
Xiaochangshu BL-27, 2, 8, 20, 26, 73, 75
Xiaogukong EX-UE-6, 46
Xiaohai SI-8, 4, 12, 37, 38, 41, 43
Xiaoluo TB-12, 2, 12, 37, 41
Xiawan CV-10, 1, 3, 13, 19, 23, 61, 63, 104
Xiaxi GB-43, 5, 6, 14, 50, 56, 57, 58
Xiguan LR-7, 11, 49, 56
Ximen PC-4, 1, 10, 37, 40, 43, 44, 143
Xingjian LR-2, 11, 49, 56, 57, 58
Xinhui GV-22, 17, 35, 61, 62
Xinshu BL-15, 2, 8, 20, 25, 73, 74, 116
Xiongxiang SP-19, 3, 11, 19, 22, 23
Xiyangguan GB-33, 5, 6, 14, 50, 54, 56
Xuanji CV-21, 1, 3, 13, 19, 23, 61, 62
Xuanli GB-6, 15, 33, 34
Xuanlu GB-5, 15, 33, 34
Xuanshu GV-5, 2, 4, 16, 20, 25, 61, 63
Xuanzhong GB-39, 5, 6, 14, 50, 56
Xuehai SP-10, 3, 11, 49, 53, 161

Yamen GV-15, 2, 16, 32, 61, 62
Yangbai GB-14, 15, 31, 33, 34, 35
Yangchi TB-4, 2, 12, 37, 43, 46
Yangfu GB-38, 5, 6, 14, 50, 56
Yanggang BL-48, 4, 8, 20, 25, 76, 77
Yanggu SI-5, 4, 12, 37, 38, 43, 46
Yangjiao GB-35, 5, 6, 14, 50, 56
Yanglao SI-6, 4, 12, 37, 38, 43
Yanglingquan GB-34, 5, 6, 14, 50, 56, 162, 163
Yangxi LI-5, 5, 6, 8, 37, 43, 46, 138, 139, 140
Yaoqi EX-B-9, 26
Yaoshu GV-2, 4, 16, 20, 26, 61, 63
Yaotongdian EX-UE-7, 46
Yaoyan EX-B-7, 26
Yaoyangguan GV-3, 2, 4, 16, 20, 26, 61, 63
Yaoyi EX-B-6, 26

Yemen TB-2, 2, 12, 37, 46
Yifeng TB-17, 32, 33, 34, 83
Yiming EX-HN-14, 33, 34, 83
Yinbai SP-1, 3, 11, 49, 56, 58
Yinbao LR-9, 11, 49, 53
Yindu KI-19, 3, 13, 19, 23, 64, 65
Yingchuang ST-16, 1, 10, 19, 23, 70, 71, 96
Yingu KI-10, 13, 48, 49, 53, 55, 56, 168
Yingxiang LI-20, 5, 6, 9, 31, 33, 34, 82, 176
Yinjiao CV-7, 1, 3, 13, 19, 24, 61, 63, 107
Yinlian LR-11, 11, 49, 53, 156
Yinlingquan SP-9, 3, 11, 49, 56
Yinmen BL-37, 2, 8, 48, 52, 158
Yinshi ST-33, 1, 10, 47, 51
Yintang EX-HN-3, 31, 35
Yinxi HT-6, 7, 37, 40, 43, 44, 149
Yishe BL-49, 4, 8, 20, 25, 76, 77
Yixi BL-45, 4, 8, 20, 25, 76, 77
Yongquan KI-1, 57
Youmen KI-21, 3, 13, 19, 23, 64, 65
Yuanye GB-22, 5, 6, 14, 21, 27, 39
Yuji LU-10, 3, 7, 37, 37, 40, 45, 152
Yunmen LU-2, 3, 7, 91
Yutang CV-18, 1, 3, 13, 19, 23, 61, 62, 96, 97
Yuyao EX-HN-4, 31
Yuzhen BL-9, 32, 33, 34
Yuzhong KI-26, 3, 13, 19, 23, 67, 68

Zhangmen LR-13, 11, 21, 22, 28
Zhaohai KI-6, 13, 49, 56, 58
Zhejin GB-23, 5, 6, 14, 21, 27, 39
Zhengying GB-17, 15, 33, 34, 35
Zhibian BL-54, 4, 8, 20, 26, 76, 78
Zhigou TB-6, 2, 12, 37, 43
Zhishi BL-52, 4, 8, 20, 26, 76, 78
Zhiyang GV-9, 2, 4, 16, 20, 25, 61, 62
Zhiyin BL-67, 4, 8, 48, 50, 56, 58
Zhizheng SI-7, 4, 12, 37, 38, 43
Zhongchong PC-9, 1, 10, 37, 40, 45
Zhongdu GB-32, 5, 6, 14, 50, 54
Zhongdu LR-6, 11, 49, 56
Zhongfeng LR-4, 11, 49, 56, 57, 58
Zhongfu LU-1, 3, 7, 178
Zhongji CV-3, 1, 3, 13, 19, 24, 61, 63, 111
Zhongkui EX-UE-4, 46
Zhongliao BL-33, 2, 8, 20, 26, 131
Zhonglüshu BL-29, 2, 8, 20, 26, 73, 75
Zhongquan EX-UE-3, 46
Zhongshu GV-7, 2, 4, 16, 20, 25, 61, 63
Zhongting CV-16, 1, 3, 13, 19, 23, 61, 62, 98
Zhongwan CV-12, 1, 3, 13, 19, 23, 61, 63, 102
Zhongzhu KI-15, 3, 13, 19, 24, 64, 66
Zhongzhu TB-3, 2, 12, 37, 46
Zhoujian EX-UE-1, 41, 43
Zhouliao LI-12, 5, 6, 8, 37, 41
Zhourong SP-20, 3, 11, 19, 22, 23, 94
Zhubin KI-9, 13, 49, 56, 168
Zigong CV-19, 1, 3, 13, 19, 23, 61, 62, 95
Zigong EX-CA-1, 29

Zulinqi GB-41, 5, 6, 14, 50, 56, 57, 58
Zuqiaoyin GB-44, 5, 6, 14, 50, 56, 57, 58

Zusanli ST-36, 1, 10, 47, 55, 164, 165, 166, 181
Zutonggu BL-66, 4, 8, 48, 50, 56, 58

Zuwuli LR-10, 11, 49, 53

ALTERNATIVE CLASSIFICATION OF EXTRAORDINARY POINTS

In this book, the classification of the names and numbers of acupuncture points conforms to that used in the National Acupuncture Points Standard of the People's Republic of China issued by the State Bureau of Technical Supervision. It is recognized that some practitioners are more familiar with the system originally used by the Shanghai College of Traditional Medicine. This alternative numbering system is listed below for the extraordinary points included in this book.

Point name	Standard [1]	Shanghai [2]	Point name	Standard [1]	Shanghai [2]
Bafeng	EX-LE-10	M-LE-8	Xiaogukong	EX-UE-6	M-UE-17
Baxie	EX-UE-9	M-UE-22	Yaoqi	EX-B-9	M-BW-29
Baichongwo	EX-LE-3	M-LE-34	Yaotongdian	EX-UE-7	M-UE-19
Bitong	n.a.	M-HN-14	Yaoyan	EX-B-7	M-BW-24
Bizhong	n.a.	M-UE-30	Yaoyi	EX-B-6	M-BW-23
Dagukong	EX-UE-5	M-UE-15	Yiming	EX-HN-14	M-HN-13
Dannang	EX-LE-6	M-LE-23	Yintang	EX-HN-3	M-HN-3
Dingchuan	EX-B-1	M-BW-1	Yuyao	EX-HN-4	M-HN-6
Erbai	EX-UE-2	M-UE-29	Zhongkui	EX-UE-4	M-UE-16
Heding	EX-LE-2	M-LE-27	Zhongquan	EX-UE-3	M-UE-33
Kuangu	EX-LE-1	M-LE-28	Zhoujian	EX-UE-1	M-UE-46
Lanwei	EX-LE-7	M-LE-13	Zigong	EX-CA-1	M-CA-18
Luozhen	n.a.	M-UE-24			
Neihuaijian	EX-LE-8	M-LE-17			
Neixiyan	EX-LE-4	M-LE-16			
Pigen	EX-B-4	M-BW-16			
Qiduan	EX-LE-12	M-LE-6			
Qiuhou	EX-HN-7	M-HN-8			
Shiqizhui	EX-B-8	M-BW-25			
Shixuan	EX-UE-11	M-UE-1			
Sifeng	EX-UE-10	M-UE-9			
Waihuaijian	EX-LE-9	M-LE-22			
Wailaogong	EX-UE-8	M-UE-23			
Weiwanxiashu (Weiguanxiashu)	EX-B-3	M-BW-12			

1. National Acupuncture Points Standard of the People's Republic of China
2. Shanghai College of Traditional Medicine